Restore Your Rest

SOLUTIONS FOR TMJ
AND SLEEP DISORDERS

Restore
your
Rest

SHAB R. KRISH
DDS, MS, DABCP, DABCDSM

Advantage®

Published by Advantage, Charleston, South Carolina.
Member of Advantage Media Group.

ADVANTAGE is a registered trademark, and the Advantage colophon is a trademark of Advantage Media Group, Inc.

Printed in the United States of America.

10 9 8 7 6 5 4 3 2 1

ISBN: 978-1-59932-883-6
LCCN: 2018953904

Cover design by Wesley Strickland.
Layout design by Megan Elger.

This publication is designed to provide accurate and authoritative information in regard to the subject matter covered. It is sold with the understanding that the publisher is not engaged in rendering legal, accounting, or other professional services. If legal advice or other expert assistance is required, the services of a competent professional person should be sought.

Advantage Media Group is proud to be a part of the Tree Neutral® program. Tree Neutral offsets the number of trees consumed in the production and printing of this book by taking proactive steps such as planting trees in direct proportion to the number of trees used to print books. To learn more about Tree Neutral, please visit **www.treeneutral.com**.

Advantage Media Group is a publisher of business, self-improvement, and professional development books and online learning. We help entrepreneurs, business leaders, and professionals share their Stories, Passion, and Knowledge to help others Learn & Grow. Do you have a manuscript or book idea that you would like us to consider for publishing? Please visit **advantagefamily.com** or call **1.866.775.1696**.

To my loving parents, and to my siblings: Mohini, Rani, Ashok, Asha, and Neelam. They have been my support and inspiration throughout my life. I'd like to thank my incredible husband, Steven Johnson, who continues to encourage me in all my endeavors. And to my children, Brittany Geeta and Alan Shaum, for always being so tolerant of my absences in pursuit of excellence.

TABLE OF CONTENTS

ABOUT THE AUTHOR

Dr. Shab Krish is passionate about helping people improve their quality of life. After suffering from temporomandibular disorder (TMD) pain herself, she began to study TMD, craniofacial pain, and sleep-disordered breathing, ultimately achieving board certifications with the American Academy of Craniofacial Pain and the American Board of Craniofacial Dental Sleep Medicine. After learning how to relieve her own pain and improve her sleep, Dr. Krish decided to devote all of her time to exclusively treating TMD, craniofacial pain, and sleep disorders by opening the TMJ & Sleep Therapy Centre of North Texas. She is also a double specialist in both periodontics and endodontics, and founder of Associates in Periodontics, Implantology & Endodontics, serving the Lewisville, Flower Mound, Denton, and surrounding North Texas communities for more than thirty years.

ACKNOWLEDGMENTS

My thanks to Dr. Steven Olmos for changing the world of dentistry and improving the quality of life for our patients with his comprehensive diagnostic and treatment protocols.

My thanks to Mr. Scott Manning for helping me and my staff achieve our personal and professional goals.

Last but not least, my sweet daughter Brittany Geeta for being the liaison between me and the editors to complete this book.

FOREWORD

It is my pleasure and honor to write this foreword to a wonderful book authored by my good friend and peer, Dr. Shab Krish.

It is a gift to be sick. That may seem like a strange thing to write, however, I feel it is accurate when your job is to help others. *I believe doctors who treat patients with the same ailments they have personally experienced can most closely relate to their patients.* I, like Dr. Krish, suffered from chronic pain and a sleep breathing disorder. I empathized as she described her search for answers to her problems, and those of her family. The frequency of these disorders is overwhelming, and in this book, she does a remarkable job explaining her journey.

I am proud that someone so skilled in her specialties and so humble to learn saw the message that I currently share and have shared for over seventeen years in the courses I teach. As she says, she was her own guinea pig and proved to herself that the protocols I have developed over the last thirty years are effective and comprehensive. We have standardized these protocols in the over forty-five TMJ & Sleep Therapy Centres located throughout seven countries.

I started teaching when I realized that if I treated patients 24/7, there would be a limited number that I could help. However, if I taught other dentists my techniques, we could give relief around the world.

The thought that a foot injury could cause facial pain is not hard to understand, as long as you are not a dentist. Any painful injury in your body will be reflected in increased facial muscle tension. The problem is that dentists are not trained in orthopedics and have an over-valued belief of dental relationships and quality of life.

Dr. Krish does a wonderful job explaining the relationships of chronic pain and breathing, in addition to what she looks for, and how she uses technology to gather data and diagnose the origin problems. Both of us are looking for the problem's origin so that long-term relief is achieved.

She shares what you should look out for, whether you are an adult or child, like how nutrition and digestion are big factors in chronic pain and skeletal dysfunction secondary to breathing disorders. Her training as an endodontist (root canal specialist) and periodontist (gum specialist) have given her a sense of understanding on why people have these problems when breathing is disordered.

I love that she shares stories of her patients that came for various reasons, and that she found a commonality that gave them an immediate solution—a way to prevent being in that situation again. *Restore Your Rest* is perfectly named.

I am so proud of Dr. Shab and her journey to now becoming board-certified in chronic pain and sleep breathing disorders. The people of North Texas are so lucky to have such a skilled clinician. All of you who read this book will be made better for the effort. She continues to give back.

Shab, congratulations on a wonderful effort!

Sincerely,

Steven R. Olmos, DDS
DABCP, DABCDSM, DAAPM, DABDSM,
FAAOP, FAACP, FICCMO, FADI, FIAO
Founder, TMJ & Sleep Therapy Centres Int'l

INTRODUCTION

A surprising number of people really open up about their lives once they're seated in the dentist's chair. That's great for me because it lets me know more about their health situation, and that gives me the chance to help them live a better life.

One patient of mine, forty-five-year-old Ann, had come in for a root canal when she opened up to me about another area of her life, one that she was initially almost too embarrassed to tell me about. "I don't even know how I can talk about it," she confided. After a little coaxing, she finally shared with me something that she had kept to herself for several months: She found out that she snored and, because she was so embarrassed about it, she no longer wanted to sleep in the same bedroom with her husband. Her husband had not a said a word; it was Ann's sister who informed her that she had a snoring problem when they had slept in the same room while taking a trip together.

"That's nothing to be embarrassed about," I assured her. But she was certain that her problems were related to age, and she was planning to have plastic surgery and other age-rejuvenating remedies to turn back the clock and stop her snoring. While aging can certainly be a factor in someone developing a snore, it is not always the primary or sole culprit. "Even babies snore," I told her. That made her laugh because, of course, who hasn't seen a soft little snore coming from a tiny baby. It may be cute, but it's also a problem, and I'll tell you why later in the book.

Then I demonstrated for Ann how easy it would be for me to fix her snore. As a child, I had perfected a "snore" while mimicking a beloved uncle. I shared that "perfect snore" with her, then quickly silenced it by moving my lower jaw forward a little. "See?" I explained. "With my jaw forward, I don't snore."

She was amazed and agreed that she need not be embarrassed. "But it is a health issue," I told her. "Snoring is often a sign that you have an obstruction in your airway making it harder for you to breathe while you sleep. By fixing your snore, you will be able to sleep better and have better health."

I performed a full examination on her and then sent her for a sleep study, which confirmed obstructive sleep apnea (OSA). I fitted her for an intraoral appliance, and she had immediate results.

Intraoral appliances are nonsurgical solutions to breathing-related sleep disorders and temporomandibular disorder (TMD). TMD is a painful disorder of the jawbone hinge, or the temporomandibular joint (TMJ). I'll talk in-depth about this disorder (which most people know as TMJ) and the solutions for it in the pages ahead.

While not everyone suffers from both sleep disorders and TMJ, there is increasing evidence that a strong connection exists between the two.[1] When you sleep, you are in what is known as a parasympathetic state, which essentially means you are completely relaxed. Your pulse rate, heart rate, and temperature are all lower than when you are awake. But if you are dealing with a sleep disorder, such as sleep-disordered breathing or sleep apnea, then periodically during the night, your body will find itself deprived of air. When that happens, your body enters into what is known as "fight-or-flight" mode—that

---

1   Steven Olmos, "Comorbidities of Chronic Facial Pain and Obstructive Sleep Apnea," *Current Opinion in Pulmonary Medicine* 22, no. 6 (November 2016): 570–75.

is the body's automatic attempt to get the air you need to live. When fight-or-flight kicks in, your brain arouses you, your heart rate increases, your jaw and neck muscles tighten, and you wake up gasping for air. Some of my patients who have gone for a sleep study have had their average normal heart rate change from 60 or 72 to 150 bpm (beats per minute). That happens while they are "sleeping." Fight-or-flight also makes your jaws move around, trying to find a position that opens your airway, which causes grinding of the teeth. And this activity happens multiple times a night—as you can imagine, it's pretty difficult to wake up refreshed when your body is fighting for your life all night.

As you can imagine, it's pretty difficult to wake up refreshed when your body is fighting for your life all night.

Yet, too often people go a long time without getting help for TMJ or a sleep disorder. Sometimes they go a lifetime without getting help. According to National Sleep Foundation estimates, some 18 million adults have OSA, and some 2 to 3 percent of children may also be affected.[2]

Part of the problem is that people who have sleep apnea may not be aware they have it, since the symptoms of TMJ and sleep disorders make these conditions difficult to diagnose. Often, to address symptoms such as a headache or restless sleep, the first solution someone will reach for is an over-the-counter pain reliever or sleep medication. Then they may seek help from numerous providers who have trouble understanding the symptoms and so are unable to provide relief.

---

2   "Obstructive Sleep Apnea," *American Association of Oral and Maxillofacial Surgeons*, accessed June 22, 2017, http://myoms.org/procedures/obstructive-sleep-apnea.

That's exactly what happened to me. You see, I suffer from TMJ and sleep apnea myself. When I first began having trouble getting good sleep, I tried to solve the problem with over-the-counter sleep aids. They helped me sleep better for a while, but I was still in pain all the time. My neck and shoulders hurt so much that I went for massages on a regular basis. "Nothing gets between me and my massage," I used to tell my staff. Without a massage, I couldn't function—it was impossible for me to see patients. I will tell you more about my journey to find relief in Chapter 1: "It's All in Your Head" and you'll see why I am able to relate to my patients' needs.

I have been a practicing periodontic and endodontic specialist for thirty years, but a few years ago, I started having a lot of pain—headaches, neck and shoulder pain, teeth clenching, and trouble sleeping. I went to several doctors, but no one seemed able to pinpoint the source of my problems. Finally, I treated myself like a patient and referred myself to dentists whose practices were focused on the treatment of TMJ disorders. But after not getting much help, I started taking classes to learn more about TMJ and sleep disorders, such as sleep-disordered breathing and sleep apnea.

While I was still in training, I found that many of my periodontic and endodontic patients had symptoms of TMJ and/or a sleep disorder. So, I began treating them and as my own skill set evolved, so did my practice.

Today, other periodontics and endodontic providers continue treating patients through my original practice, Associates in Periodontics, Implantology & Endodontics. But my passion for TMJ and sleep inspired me to start a completely new practice, TMJ & Sleep Therapy Centre of North Texas, where I focus solely on TMJ and sleep disorders.

In the chapters ahead, I will share with you more about TMJ and sleep-disordered breathing, including sleep apnea. I will discuss how TMJ and sleep disorders are diagnosed and treated, and how that treatment is customized to each patient's needs. There is a chapter on sleep apnea in kids—it's not just a condition that affects adults. I'll also discuss measures for preventing sleep disorders, including both structural and functional changes that can be made earlier in life along with the role of food in TMJ and sleep for adults.

I've included a number of actual patient stories in this book, but to protect their privacy, I've included only first or fictional names. Through these stories and the knowledge that I'm sharing, I hope you will see that by addressing the issues of TMJ and sleep disorders, we're helping people live better—we're changing their lives.

CHAPTER 1

"IT'S ALL IN YOUR HEAD"

*"Of course it is happening inside your head, Harry, but
why on earth should that mean that it is not real?"*

—J.K. ROWLING, *Harry Potter and the Deathly Hallows*

When my daughter graduated from high school, my family came to stay for a while to celebrate her achievement. My best friend and her husband were the first in the family to arrive, so I gave them the choice of bedrooms—upstairs or down.

In making her choice, my best friend simply requested "the room that has access to a couch."

"Why a couch?" I asked.

She explained that, on a nightly basis, her snoring wakes her husband and when he can't get back to sleep because she is so noisy, he gets up and goes to the couch in the other room. That's where he regularly finishes his last few hours of sleep.

Hearing of my best friend's plight, I knew I could help, so during her stay, I performed a cursory exam that showed she likely had a sleep disorder and TMJ, a dysfunction of the jaw joint and muscles. Because she was only in town for a short time, I advised her to have a sleep study performed when she returned home.

Back home in Wisconsin, she requested a sleep study from her family physician, who told her she didn't need one. "You can't have sleep apnea," he said. "You're female, you're thin. You're not someone who should have sleep apnea." Since sleep apnea has long been a problem associated primarily with overweight men, and my best friend is generally underweight, there was the assumption that she could not be afflicted with it.

That was an unacceptable answer to me. She continued to insist that she needed to be tested, until her primary physician relented and prescribed a polysomnography (PSG), or sleep study. At the sleep lab, the technicians attached sensors to her that let them monitor her sleep from a separate room. The results of the PSG revealed that she did have moderate sleep apnea.

She came back to my office, where I conducted a full examination on her, checking her mouth, nose, jaws, and head and neck muscles. In addition to sleep apnea, I found that she did have dysfunction in her temporomandibular joint (TMJ). We fitted her with an intraoral appliance designed to treat both her sleep apnea and her TMJ. She wears the appliance nightly, and it has resolved her snoring along with other problems she did not even know she had, including teeth clenching and disrupted sleep. She sleeps through the night now—and her husband no longer spends his nights on the couch!

My best friend's situation is not uncommon. Men, in particular, often tell me, "I snore, but it doesn't bother me. In fact, I sleep really well. But my snoring bothers my wife to the point that she's kicked me out of the bedroom. Can you help me get back in?" I call this *secondary snoring*, where one bed partner is affected by the other's snoring. No matter who is snoring, it's a bad sign—snoring is a sign that something is wrong.

Snoring and sleep disorders are so commonly associated with overweight men that the issue has earned the nicknamed the "Pickwickian syndrome." Named after the sleepy, overweight, red-faced boy described by Charles Dickens in his novel *The Pickwick Papers*, Pickwickian syndrome, formally known as obesity hypoventilation syndrome (OHS), is a breathing disorder experienced by some obese people. The disorder is the result of a buildup of carbon dioxide in the blood, which happens when the person's weight affects their breathing to the point that they don't get enough oxygen. People with OHS often have obstructive sleep apnea (OSA).

Because weight is one factor causing sleep apnea, anyone—not just men—can experience it, even women and children.

Now, before I go any further, let me clarify a bit of terminology. Most people have heard of the term *TMJ* and use it to refer to pain in the jaw area. TMJ stands for temporomandibular joint, which is the "hinge" that connects your jaw to your skull. When a person experiences pain or tenderness in the jaw area, they are actually suffering from what is known as temporomandibular disorder, or *TMD*. Since most people are more familiar with the term TMJ than they are with TMD, I will use the term TMJ throughout the rest of the book to discuss the disorder of the temporomandibular joint.

A couple of other terms to clarify include *sleep-disordered breathing* and *sleep apnea*. Sleep-disordered breathing refers to a range of conditions that affect sleep; sleep apnea is one of those conditions. As a board-certified diplomate of the American Academy of Craniofacial Pain and the American Board of Craniofacial Dental Sleep Medicine of the American Academy of Craniofacial Pain, I am trained and qualified to treat sleep-disordered breathing and sleep apnea. However, while I can treat sleep apnea, the diagnosis for sleep apnea can only be made by a sleep physician. That happens following a sleep study, which takes specific measurements in order to determine the severity of the sleep apnea.

In the pages ahead, I will sometimes refer to sleep-disordered breathing and sleep apnea as sleep disorders or breathing-related sleep disorders. I will also discuss the connection between TMJ and sleep apnea in more depth in the chapters ahead. For now, let me share with you a bit about my own journey to find answers for TMJ and sleep apnea. I think you'll see why I can empathize with patients.

MANY PROVIDERS, NO SOLUTIONS

My best friend's situation in not being able to get answers from her primary care provider is also a common problem for many other people. Many people seek help from different providers, but fail to find relief for their symptoms. Too often, patients are told a problem is "all in their head," when the problems are very real.

Yes, TMJ and sleep disorders are physically "all in your head," or almost anyway. The problems associated with TMJ and breathing-related sleep disorders are in your mouth, and your jaws, and your airway, and maybe even in your neck and shoulders. If you don't do something about the problems, then they can affect other areas of the body as well. In short, if your body is telling you that something is wrong, then you must listen and get help.

Take it from someone who knows: I was like many people who experience pain that was ultimately found to be the result of TMJ and sleep apnea. My problems started after I lost my retainers that I wore following treatment with braces. Those retainers actually consisted of a night guard to protect my upper teeth and a wire retainer on my lower teeth.

When I sought replacement retainers, I was given a night guard for my lower teeth and a wire retainer for my upper teeth. Unfortunately, the replacement retainers did not really work as well as my original retainers.

I began snoring at night and wasn't sleeping well. When I did sleep, I would wake in the morning with pain in my neck and shoulders. I turned to over-the-counter pain and sleep aids for relief, but within only a few days of taking the medication, my body grew accustomed to it—it no longer worked.

Over time, the lack of sleep at night and the pain upon waking really began to affect my ability to function well. I told my husband: "If I could only sleep at night, I could perform better during the day." (That's the same phrase I hear often from my patients today.) I could make it through the day as long as I drank a lot of coffee and focused on work. But whenever there was downtime, I'd focus on the pain. At the end of the day, I was exhausted. If I was able to make it to a workout, I was completely worn out when I was done, and no matter how often I went to the gym, I kept putting on weight.

I turned to another provider for solutions, and he prescribed a muscle relaxer that was so strong I could only take it on Saturdays. It took all day Sunday for the initial effects to wear off, but by Monday morning I was able to function very well. In fact, the medication gave me relief for nearly a week at a time until, once again, my body grew accustomed to it. Then, by midweek, I found myself turning to other over-the-counter pain relievers again. During that time, it was common to see me holding hot coffee mugs against my face just to relieve the chronic pain.

During that time, it was common to see me holding hot coffee mugs against my face just to relieve the chronic pain.

Finally, I decided that if I were going to find a solution to my problems, then I needed to treat myself as if I were one of my own patients. I began researching solutions when I came upon providers who knew about both TMJ and sleep disorders. I found one who gave me an appliance that had to be worn twenty-four hours a day. When I first put the appliance in, I drove the twenty minutes to my office and by the time I got there I was so happy—I felt great! The appliance was working. I thought I was returning to my former, pain-free self.

Unfortunately, that appliance only worked for a couple of days before the pain came back—with a vengeance. Undeterred, I continued to look for answers. After all, I was in pain and I needed to function—I had to get to the root of the problem. Finally, I asked one of the doctors where I, an endodontist and periodontist, could learn more about TMJ treatment myself. He referred me to the American Academy of Craniofacial Pain (AACP).

Through the AACP, I began taking courses primarily on TMJ. I was actually a "guinea pig" for some of the lessons because I was suffering from the same problems the other doctors were learning about. The program also required participants to go through a sleep study, which diagnosed me with mild sleep apnea. When those results came back, one AACP instructor suggested I try a combination appliance for TMJ and sleep apnea. Unfortunately, like one of my earlier appliances, it forced me to sleep with my mouth slightly ajar, which caused me to wake every day with dry mouth even though I was drooling at the same time. I asked for the appliance to be altered so that I could close my mouth, but then my jaw started locking—four times I had a locked jaw that had to be massaged until it released.

The AACP courses gave me a good foundation on the basics of treating TMJ, but as a "newbie," I was admittedly a little confused. There was a lot of information and many different approaches to treatment. Each instructor had a solution, and they all appeared to work, depending on the patient's situation.

While in those courses, I decided to become an AACP Fellow, which required me to have two hundred continuing education (CE) credits. Since the program I was in only conferred one hundred credits, I asked the AACP chairman about a good resource for the remaining credits and he mentioned Steven Olmos, founder of TMJ & Sleep Therapy Centre International in San Diego.

The initial courses only covered TMJ, they did not cover sleep disorders, which, as I would learn from Dr. Olmos, were two extremely connected issues. That's one reason patients don't get proper treatment. Too many dentists and doctors are treating only one of the causes—they're not addressing the connection between TMJ and breathing-related sleep disorders.

I was actually on my way to San Diego for my first class in Dr. Olmos's program when my jaw locked. On my arrival in San Diego, Dr. Olmos examined me and found that my bite was so misaligned because of muscle spasms that I needed a cold laser treatment before an impression of my teeth could even be made. Ultimately, through Dr. Olmos's exams and a sleep study, it was discovered that I had TMJ and sleep apnea. He made me an appliance to be worn during the day and another to wear as I slept, and together, those resolved my pain.

Through Dr. Olmos's program, I really began to see the connections between TMJ and sleep disorders. The comprehensive training covered everything from anatomy and pharmacology to physiology and neurology, which gave me great insights into how the two disorders affect the whole body. I also learned various treatments for solving patients' problems, and Dr. Olmos's protocol is what we use in my practice today. By being part of Dr. Olmos's TMJ & Sleep Therapy Centre International, we're able to bring patients his newest discoveries, latest technologies, and ever-improving protocols.

The more I learned, the more I began to recognize the symptoms in patients—and I was amazed at how many had symptoms of both TMJ and sleep disorders. In fact, the first patient I treated with Dr. Olmos's protocol was a woman who, while undergoing a gum graft, asked me to give her a shot of anesthetic in her jaw to ease her pain, a common but only temporary treatment for TMJ. I did not administer that shot, but instead made an appliance that helped her TMJ. My second patient had a similar situation—he was in for other dental work and asked if I could help alleviate his jaw pain.

Before long, I was getting referrals from other dentists, and some patients were even driving several hours for treatment. One of those patients was Rose, who drove three hours from Austin. After treatment with day and night appliances, she told me, "Dr. Krish, you've changed the quality of my life. I used to be so miserable all the time, and now I'm like a real person. I'm pleasant again." That was something I never heard from patients when I was doing grafts, implants, and root canals.

After I had finished my two hundred credit hours, and simultaneously treated twenty-five patients, I became an AACP Fellow and I began to look at what that meant for my practice.

A NEW DIRECTION

Throughout my journey to find relief, I was met with many of the same obstacles and comments as I hear from my patients, from trying solutions that provide no relief, to nearly being denied treatment because of insurance limitations, to being told my problems were "all in my head." Because I'm a dentist, I also encountered the perception that I would be a challenging patient simply because of my medical knowledge.

Since I was seeing so many patients who had both TMJ and sleep disorders, and I saw a void in solutions for them, I decided to move full time into treating the two conditions. Until recently, I had two practices, but I have since sold the one that offers periodontics, implants, and endodontics. It remains next door, however, in the same building, and it is complementary to the work I currently do. The other practice is where my passion now lies. That practice is the TMJ & Sleep Therapy Centre of North Texas, which focuses solely on TMJ and sleep disorders.

Today, it gives me great pleasure to be able to help people dealing with problems associated with TMJ and sleep disorders.

Now let's delve into some of the nitty-gritty about these two conditions: TMJ and sleep disorders.

CHAPTER 2

TMJ AND SLEEP APNEA — THE MORE YOU KNOW

"I'm dying from the treatment of too many physicians."

—ALEXANDER THE GREAT

Before becoming a patient of mine, Tara had been suffering from headaches and neck pain for years and had been to numerous health care providers trying to get relief. As a pharmaceutical sales representative, she carried around big bags of samples, which she thought was the cause of her pain. When the problem reached the point that her arms were starting to feel numb, she finally switched to smaller bags. Unfortunately, that did not solve her problems.

Still dealing with pain on a daily basis, she went to a physician, who sent her to a neurologist. The neurologist thought physical therapy was the best solution, so Tara's next consult was with a physical therapist. While physical therapy provided some relief, Tara still had a lot of pain in the long run. Even when she offered up her own best-guess about the problem, one provider failed to see a connection.

"My face hurts because I'm clenching and grinding. Could it be TMJ?" she asked.

But the provider simply replied: "What does TMJ have to do with your neck pain?"

Finally, when Tara broke a tooth, she went to her dentist, who immediately identified TMJ as the culprit. Fortunately, her dentist referred Tara to me.

We conducted a complete range of tests and confirmed that she had TMJ. Before I prepared her an appliance for TMJ, I suggested that she also undergo a sleep study since I could tell from my initial exam that she had an obstructed airway and was likely also dealing with a sleep disorder. Although the treatments I offer can relieve sleep disorders, sleep apnea can only be diagnosed by a sleep physician who interprets the results of a sleep study. Since the costs of seeing so many providers were beginning to add up, and she had a family member dealing with a life-threatening disease, she could no longer afford to take more time off work. Tara turned down the sleep study. So, I went ahead and created an appliance to treat only her TMJ.

Finally, when Tara broke a tooth, she went to her dentist, who immediately identified TMJ as the culprit. Fortunately, her dentist referred Tara to me.

After she used the TMJ appliance for a short time, she happily reported that she felt better than she had in years. The numbness in her arm went away, and she was feeling better overall.

About a year later, Tara came back to see me and was in a better place to have the sleep study done. The results? Tara had moderate sleep apnea.

The fix then was fairly easy—all we had to do was convert her existing TMJ appliance into a combo appliance that would also address her sleep apnea. But when I told her we needed to have her

TMJ appliance for a few days to make the conversion, she adamantly refused: "There's no way I'll part with this appliance," she said. Prior to having the sleep study, she had been required to leave the appliance out for three days, which she said were the most miserable days she'd had in a long time. So, instead of converting the existing appliance, we had a new appliance made that addressed both her TMJ and sleep apnea.

There is a very real connection between TMJ and sleep apnea—80 percent of TMJ patients have sleep issues, and 75 percent of sleep apnea patients have TMJ.[3] Yet even though the two are often connected, one condition does not necessarily cause the other. Unfortunately, TMJ and sleep apnea can go undiagnosed—sometimes for years. In Tara's case, it definitely was true—and it was costly. She had seen five providers before coming to see me.

Besides the fact that TMJ and sleep disorders are difficult to diagnose, there are a number of reasons people don't get treated for years.

For instance, people often assume that snoring is a condition that occurs as a natural part of aging. Others just ignore it; they don't recognize it as a symptom of a sleep disorder. Some just choose to overlook the situation; a snoring spouse or partner may make it hard to get a good night's sleep, but they just accept the snoring as a part of life. But it is never okay to snore. Snoring usually means that the airway is partially blocked. That means a reduced amount of air is being breathed in. Any discussion on the subject of snoring is usually unpleasant because it is common for people who snore to not even know they do, and to deny it when it is pointed out to them. Finally, when the spouse or partner can no longer tolerate the noise, the snorer

3   A.E. Sanders et al., "Sleep Apnea Symptoms and Risk of Temporomandibular Disorder," *Journal of Dental Research* 92, no. 7 (July 2013): S70–S77, https://doi.org/10.1177/0022034513488140

will come to see me for an evaluation. Many husbands are motivated to come to us because the wife has kicked them out of the bedroom.

Often, snorers don't really believe they snore. But once I start asking questions during a consultation, such as "Do you wake up refreshed?" the snorers start to recognize they might have a problem.

Similarly, people with TMJ often know they have a problem, but they don't know the source of it until someone else points out symptoms, such as grinding the teeth at night. As I mentioned in the previous chapter, a deeper explanation about TMJ is in order.

TMJ DISORDER (TMD)

The TMJ is a hinge connecting your jawbone, or mandible, to your skull. Specifically, the TMJ connects with your temporal bone, which is located on the lower side of your skull. In between the jawbone and skull there is a disc made of cartilage that is held in place by facial ligaments and muscles. That disc acts as a cushion to keep the bones from rubbing against each other when you move your jaw to talk, chew, swallow, or yawn. The whole system is similar to the ball and socket joints in your body, like your shoulder, for instance. When everything functions correctly, the muscles and ligaments around the jawbone work together to make jaw movement smooth and pain free.

The whole system is similar to the ball and socket joints in your body, like your shoulder, for instance.

When the area is affected by pain or tenderness, it is suffering from a dysfunction that also involves the surrounding facial tissues. TMJ can cause severe pain when you try to open your mouth wide, and can even cause the jaw to catch or lock in the open or closed position. The pain or tenderness that you feel in your jaw area can occur at the joint in front of the ear, or in the head, neck, and shoulders. Sometimes the pain only occurs when the jaw is used, and sometimes the pain lingers.

SYMPTOMS THAT MAY INDICATE TMJ INCLUDE:

- pain when chewing jaw sounds: popping, clicking, grating, or crepitus
- bruxism: clenching and grinding
- pain or numbness in lower jaw
- difficulty opening the mouth
- frequent migraines/headaches
- ear pain, congestion, ringing
- facial pain
- neck/back/shoulder pain

Early symptoms of TMJ often include a clicking or popping sound in the jaw area. The clicking, popping and jaw locking happen when the disc is displaced and moves around on the condyle, or the end portion of the jawbone that fits into the concave or bowl-like "socket" area in the skull. Instead of staying in place to act as a cushion, the disc moves forward (anterior/medial) when you open or close your mouth. Often, these earliest symptoms are ignored or overlooked since they seem to resolve on their own or come and go.

The center of the disc does not contain nerve endings, so when it is in place and functioning as it should, then you won't have pain in your jaw area. But when it gets displaced, then the retrodiscal tissues, which are located behind the joint, get pulled forward and compressed. These tissues do contain nerve endings and blood supply, but they are not meant to take the pressure of chewing and swallowing—that's the disc's role. When the tissue's nerve endings are compressed, they let you know it by causing you pain.

Jaw locking occurs when the disc jumps forward (anterior/medial) off the end of the condyle because the ligament has stretched to the point that it allows that degree of displacement. A displaced disc can even worsen to the point that it's difficult to fully open the jaw; you may literally have to massage and/or reposition your jaw a bit so you can open your mouth wider. The disc can even cause a person's mouth to lock in the closed position. When that happens, the disc is dislocated in *front* of the condyle, and prevents the jaw from opening wide. It must be massaged back in place in order to open the mouth.

Displacement of the Articular Disc

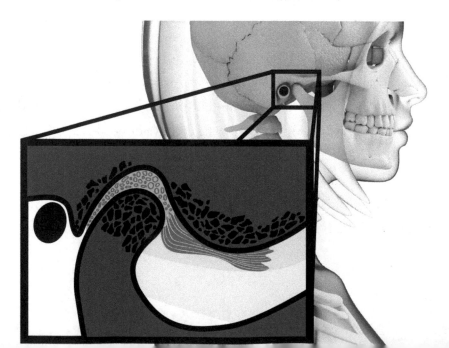

Ultimately, the symptoms of clicking, popping, and pain worsen until you experience *crepitus*, a "sandy" or grinding feeling when opening and closing your mouth.

The disc can displace for any number of reasons. The ligament can be stretched when you hold your mouth open for a long period of time, such as when undergoing a procedure at the dentist's office, or when you open wide in order to be intubated for anesthesia when undergoing a medical procedure.

Since the jaw and disc ligaments involved in TMJ are also attached to the bone inside the ear, it's common for people to think that their ears are somehow the problem. Symptoms of TMJ also include ear pain, itchiness, or stuffiness, or even tinnitus (ringing in the ears). Often, a person will go to an ear, nose, and throat specialist (ENT) because they think they are having ear trouble when the problem is actually TMJ.

TMJ symptoms also include clenching or grinding at night, a condition known as bruxism. Bruxism can lead to frequent headaches and even migraines because of the chronic pressure that is applied to the bones and muscles. That pain can migrate to the neck, shoulders, and back. Bruxism can also injure the facial ligaments by applying constant pressure that causes them to stretch and tighten. Once the ligament has been stretched, it can become susceptible to additional injury. When I see evidence of dental changes in a person's mouth— teeth that are worn down or broken—I know that I'm probably looking at someone who clenches their jaws or grinds their teeth at night.

Clenching and grinding are secondary to sleep-related arousals that result in rhythmic muscle activity. Bruxism is actually related to the arousals that occur during sleep as a result of the body's attempt to open the airway. That is where TMJ can be linked to sleep disorders.

The airway relaxes at night when a person sleeps. When a person is dealing with a sleep disorder, their jaw muscles may clench in an effort to keep the airway open.

While these are the most common symptoms of TMJ, left undiagnosed and treated, TMJ can ultimately affect other areas of the body that do not appear to be related. That was the case with Tara—the numbness in her arm was ultimately a symptom of her TMJ.

Now, some symptoms of TMJ overlap with those of sleep disorders. Let's take a closer look at sleep-disordered breathing and sleep apnea and some of the symptoms that may indicate either of these is present.

SLEEP-DISORDERED BREATHING AND SLEEP APNEA

As I mentioned, sleep apnea is one form of sleep-disordered breathing. Sleep-disordered breathing (SDB) is a group of disorders involving difficulty breathing that can disrupt your sleep. These can range from occasional or mild snoring to Upper Airway Resistance Syndrome (UARS) caused by a partial blockage of the air passage. As I mentioned earlier, I often refer to these as sleep-related breathing disorders or sleep disorders.

Sleep apnea, on the other hand, is a serious condition that, left untreated, can increase your risk of having a heart attack or stroke, or can lead to irregular heartbeat, high blood pressure, heart disease, and decreased libido.[4] Some 26 percent of Americans are at a high risk for sleep apnea.[5] And yet sleep apnea is so misunderstood that doctors and dentists worldwide are giving patients anesthesia without

---

4   "Obstructive Sleep Apnea," American Association of Oral and Maxillofacial Surgeons.

5   Olmos, "Comorbidities of Chronic Facial Pain."

recognizing or addressing the issue. They're putting their patients to sleep, a state in which they literally stop breathing, without truly understanding their health situation.

Apnea is a pause in breathing for ten seconds or longer. Hypopnea is a partial loss of air lasting for ten seconds or longer.

Later in the book, I'll talk more about the sleep tests. These give the Apnea-Hypopnea Index (AHI), a number used to indicate the severity of sleep apnea. It is calculated by finding the number of apnea events divided by the amount of time slept.[6]

There are two kinds of sleep apnea: central sleep apnea (CSA) and obstructive sleep apnea (OSA). CSA involves the central nervous system and is caused when the brain simply stops sending signals to the muscles that control breathing—your brain stops telling you to take a breath. CSA may occur alongside OSA, but it is often associated with more serious conditions, such as congestive heart failure, hypothyroid disease, Alzheimer's disease, or Parkinson's. OSA is the most common form of sleep apnea and is caused by an obstruction of the airway.

Of the two types—OSA and CSA—OSA can be easier to control since it involves removing the obstruction. I'll talk more about how sleep apnea is diagnosed and treated in the next two chapters. For now, let's look at some of the causes of OSA.

A number of conditions can cause the obstruction of air. One of the main conditions involves the nares (nostrils or nasal passages). When the nasal passages are blocked for some reason, naturally, it is harder to breathe. Those reasons might include a collapse of the nasal passages, a deviated septum (a displaced nasal passage), polyps (a

---

6   "Understanding the Results: Sleep Apnea," *Harvard Medical School*, September 5, 2014, accessed at http://healthysleep.med.harvard.edu/sleep-apnea/diagnosing-osa/understanding-results

fleshy growth), or swelling—all of these can prevent air from travelling through the airway to the lungs. The nasal passages are part of the respiratory system, those parts of the body that involve breathing and include everything from the nose and mouth to the lungs. The nasal passages are part of what is known as the upper respiratory system, which are the parts of your body from your face through your neck that are involved in breathing. When any part of that system—such as a nasal passage—is blocked, it reduces your ability to get enough air or oxygen into your body. It's a bit like a garden hose; the size of the hose and its collapsibility determines the amount of water that flows through it. The smaller the hose and the more collapsible, the less water available for your garden. Similarly, the smaller the airway, the less air you are able to get to your lungs where you need it. Correcting a blockage opens up the hose (nasal passage) wide and allows for better airflow. As we get older, the muscles lose their tonus and the airway can become more collapsible.

Often, other areas of your upper respiratory system are obstructed. For instance, your airway can be blocked by tonsils, adenoids, sagging palate (tissue roof of the mouth), and the uvula, which is that funny-looking pendulum of flesh that hangs down at the back of your throat. The tongue can also cause airway obstruction, especially if you have a large tongue or if it rests at the back of your throat. Even soft tissue at the back of your throat can cause obstruction. That can happen if the tissue loses muscle tone or increases in size due to excess weight or obesity.

SYMPTOMS THAT MAY INDICATE A SLEEP DISORDER OR SLEEP APNEA:

- loud snoring

- excessive daytime sleepiness

- poor nighttime sleeping

- nighttime waking episodes

- morning headaches

- teeth grinding and dental changes

- dry mouth and a chronic need for water at night

- neck and shoulder pain

- depression

- diabetes

- obesity

- heartburn and GERD

Snoring, as I've mentioned, can indicate sleep-disordered breathing or sleep apnea. Snoring happens even when the airway is only partially blocked, for instance, by the uvula or excess tissue. The sound actually occurs when the uvula and tissue vibrate as you breathe in and out. Loud snoring—which we've heard some spouses and partners of our patients describe as "a freight train going by"—is caused when you try to breathe in a lot of air through a very small opening, an airway that is very small or constricted.

When someone suffers from a sleep disorder, they generally do not wake up in the morning feeling rested and refreshed. That seems a given for someone who has been through a night of waking events. If you wake up thinking you need another hour or two of sleep, then chances are you had a number of waking episodes during the night that disrupted the sleep cycle. The sleep cycle is basically four stages that the body goes through during sleep, from falling to sleep to very deep sleep. The body needs that deep sleep to regenerate the brain and nourish the body. The ability to learn, for instance, is one benefit of getting at least seven hours of sleep per night. While you are awake, information is taken in and stored in a part of the brain known as the hippocampus. However, the hippocampus has limited capacity for storing information and after about sixteen hours, the brain as a whole has had enough—it will not function after being awake that long. During sleep, the hippocampus essentially turns short-term memories stored during the waking hours into learned information.[7] That allows memories to be recalled later. Studies have found that time spent sleeping, versus time awake, has a 20 to 40 percent greater impact on the ability to retain memories.[8] That percentage is greatest during the early hours of sleep, known as the non-rapid eye movement (NREM) part of the sleep cycle.[9] That is even true when the NREM part of the sleep cycle occurs during a short nap, which is why naps, for some people, are so rejuvenating.

Daytime sleepiness is another potential symptom of a sleep disorder. After a night of disrupted sleep, it's common to periodically nod off, which can lead to an accident while driving. Accidents caused by drowsy drivers are not solely caused by people falling asleep at the wheel. They are also caused when someone is so sleep deprived that they essentially nod off for a brief instant; they enter what is known as a "microsleep," during which the brain basically shuts down for just an instant—even a couple of seconds of microsleep is long enough to cause an accident.[10] One study even compared

---

7   Matthew Walker, *Why We Sleep by Doctor: Unlocking the Power of Sleep and Dreams* (New York: Scribner, 2017).

8   Ibid.

9   Ibid.

10   Ibid.

drowsy driving to driving drunk and found that individuals with only four hours of sleep were as impaired as individuals who had eight hours of sleep but were legally drunk.[11] Daytime sleepiness can also lead to lost productivity on the job, and it can even affect your personal relationships.

Having a dry mouth upon waking is another potential symptom of a sleep disorder. A dry mouth is the result of breathing with the mouth open all night, which is another way the body automatically fights for air when it encounters an obstruction in the airway. The problem with chronic mouth breathing is that it can eventually cause dental problems, such as gingivitis and gum disease, because the body needs saliva to control bacteria in the mouth.

GERD, or acid reflux, can occur with a sleep disorder. GERD results from the body applying extra pressure to the abdomen area in its efforts to catch a breath. That can then push acid out of the stomach and into the mouth, which can then potentially affect the teeth. A 2006 US National Health and Wellness Survey found that patients with GERD had more than twice the likelihood of experiencing sleep difficulties.[12] Sleep disorders can also cause gastrointestinal (GI) disorders, or it can worsen existing GI symptoms.

Obesity and sleep disorders go hand in hand to create a truly vicious cycle. When you sleep, your body produces certain hormones that help your body to function. Two of these regulate your appetite: ghrelin makes you feel hungry, leptin tells you when you are full. If you don't get adequate amounts of sleep, your body does not produce leptin in the proper quantities, so you feel hungry all the time. One study found that cravings for higher-calorie foods, sweets, carbohy-

---

11   Ibid.

12   Reema Mody et al., "Effects of Gastroesophageal Reflux Disease on Sleep and Outcomes," *Clinical Gastroenterology and Hepatology* 7, no. 9 (2009): 953–59.

drates, and salty snacks were 30 to 40 percent higher when a person is sleep deprived.[13] Unless you have a lot of willpower, you will give in to those feelings of hunger more often than you should. That adds weight. When you add more weight, your neck increases in size.

Women should have a neck size no greater than 16 inches, for men 17 inches is maximum. Beyond those measurements, the neck begins to add excess fat tissue and can begin crowding the airway, compounding existing sleep disorders or creating sleep apnea. People also tend to gain weight from sleep disorders because they get up at night more frequently and head to the refrigerator for a snack. Lack of sleep also makes a person less apt to exercise—without sleep, who wants to go to the gym after work? Before I began having TMJ and sleep apnea problems, I was an exercise fiend. I would go to the gym every day after work and get in a good workout. When my TMJ and sleep apnea left me exhausted, I would go home after work, sit down and eat, and call it a day. I, too, was stuck in that vicious cycle.

As I mentioned earlier, untreated sleep apnea raises the risk of developing heart disease or having a stroke. A study of millions of men and women around the world reported in 2011 found that, within seven to twenty-five years of the launch of the study, those with progressively shortened periods of sleep had a 45 percent higher incidence of death from heart disease.[14] Another study found that sleep's impact on heart disease continued even after other risk factors, such as smoking, lack of exercise, and excess weight, were controlled.[15] The link, it appears, is in the amount of calcification in the arteries that supply the heart with blood. A study by the University of Chicago found that people sleeping five to six hours per night,

---

13   Walker, *Why We Sleep*.

14   Ibid.

15   Ibid.

compared to those sleeping seven to eight hours, had 200 to 300 percent more calcification.[16]

Sleep deprivation has been found to increase the size of cancer tumors. According to a study in mice, cancer was more aggressive and spread to surrounding tissues and bone in the mice in the study that were deprived of sleep.[17] In fact, the immune system, as a whole, functions better when a person gets enough regular, deep sleep.

Another hormone that dysfunctions without adequate sleep is vasopressin, which concentrates urine so the bladder doesn't send a signal to the brain to wake you up to go to the bathroom. Now, it's one thing to drink water too close to bedtime and then have to get up later to go. But too often, as people age, they reach the point where it seems normal to get up multiple times at night to go to the bathroom. It's not normal. When your sleep is disrupted by a sleep disorder, so is your body's production of vasopressin.

Other hormones that are disrupted when you don't get adequate sleep include growth hormone, which children need to grow and which helps an aging body heal.

Production of melatonin, the sleep hormone, is also disrupted. Melatonin is released into the body as it begins to get dark. Here again, it's a cycle—when you don't sleep you don't produce enough melatonin, and without melatonin, you don't sleep.

Melatonin regulates the timing of sleep, but not the generation of sleep.[18] Natural production of the hormone melatonin begins at dusk and then decreases by dawn. While taking a melatonin supplement may help signal to the body that it's time to sleep, it does not

---

16   Ibid.
17   Ibid.
18   Ibid.

deepen sleep or make for better sleep. Yet melatonin supplements are commonly taken and even prescribed to children.

Sleep disorders can also raise levels of the stress hormone, cortisol, which can wreak havoc on your body. Overproduction of cortisol happens when your body enters the "fight-or-flight" state in its effort to get the air it needs. Your body also produces more cortisol when you have TMJ pain, because aching jaws raise your stress level. As part of a patient's overall assessment we take photos, and when a person has too much cortisol it shows—their eyes are so big they look like they're caught in the headlights of a car. Too much cortisol can also keep you up at night, which as I mentioned can lead to weight gain. And it can cause blood glucose levels to rise, potentially putting you in danger of developing diabetes.

Ultimately, too much cortisol can contribute to feelings of depression. A person dealing with chronic pain may end up feeling depressed, in part because they just get tired of not feeling well, in part because they can't seem to get answers for their problems. Sometimes, they will be prescribed an antidepressant, but that can actually make the situation worse. Some antidepressants can cause a person to grind their teeth, some actually lead to insomnia. Studies have even found a link between lack of sleep and suicidal thoughts and acts in adolescents.[19]

TMJ and sleep disorders can be difficult to diagnose because the symptoms are so insidious; they start out subtly and can seem very vague or minor at first. But as the problems worsen, so do the symptoms, until the pain becomes chronic. In some ways, it's a vicious cycle because pain anywhere in the body can make it difficult to get a good night's sleep, leading to sleep disorders and possibly TMJ.

---

19 Ibid.

Quality of life depends on getting good sleep, and that relies on being able to breathe. When a person is able to breathe well, and they get good sleep, they live longer and have a healthier life. That's the goal of being informed about TMJ and sleep disorders—to live long and healthy.

Now let's look at some of the ways TMJ and sleep disorders are diagnosed.

CHAPTER 3

DIAGNOSING TMJ AND SLEEP DISORDERS

"Diagnosis is not the end but the beginning of practice."

—MARTIN H. FISCHER

When I was taking classes in California to learn more about TMJ and sleep disorders, I mentioned to Dr. Olmos that my TMJ appliance did not seem to be working. I was still having a lot of neck pain, so I asked him to take a look.

He checked my TMJ and the appliance and determined that everything was working as it should. Seemingly unrelated, I was also beginning to have pain in my feet. The pain wasn't that bad at the time, but over the next few months it began to get increasingly worse until I could no longer walk properly. Back in Texas, I went to a podiatrist, a foot doctor, who diagnosed the problem as heel spurs. Impressions were made of my feet so that I could have custom shoe inserts made to relieve the pain.

Since the inserts had to be specially made for me, the doctor wrapped my feet with tape to help alleviate the pain until I had the inserts in hand. The tape was very snug, but it felt great! Right away I was able to put my shoes on and walk again. I left her office and headed to the airport, on my way to another TMJ/sleep-disordered breathing class in California. When I took my seat on the plane, I also realized that for the first time in a while, I was able to turn my head side-to-side without feeling any pain in my neck. I was amazed: not only was my foot pain gone, but some of my TMJ symptoms had also disappeared.

The class in San Diego was held at a hotel located on the beach. For the first two days of my trip, I felt great because the tape was still wrapped around my feet. It had loosened a little when it got wet while I was in the shower, but for the most part, it was still holding and doing its job.

I was scheduled to leave on the afternoon of the third day, so that morning I was determined to take a walk on the beach and let my toes feel the sand and surf. I carefully unwrapped the tape so that I could put it back on after my walk. Then I went out to walk on the beach. Unfortunately, my walk was cut short because, unbelievably, my pain returned.

Back in my room, I found that I could not get the tape wrapped snugly enough to relieve the pain as it had before. So I visited a local drugstore and found some compression sleeves that fit over my feet and heels—that pretty much did the trick.

With Dr. Olmos's diagnosis, and the aid of my podiatrist, my TMJ is no longer causing me pain in my neck—or my feet. Fixing my foot problem took care of my neck problem. But it took that extra digging into my condition to pinpoint the problems one at a time and then find solutions.

It's like the song we used to sing as children, "Dem Bones." There's actually truth to those lyrics. Since all the structures of the body are connected, the source of pain may actually be caused by a problem somewhere else in the body. In my case, I was clenching because of the problems with my feet, and that clenching was causing problems in my neck.

My experience demonstrates the importance of delving into each patient's health history to help get to the root of the problem.

THE HEALTH HISTORY

An accurate diagnosis is the key to an effective treatment plan. That begins by taking a deep look into the patient's health history.

At the TMJ & Sleep Therapy Centre of North Texas, the first consult begins by having the patient fill out a twelve-page intake form. The questions on the form are designed to uncover any unresolved issues the patient may be experiencing. It asks about things such as:

- symptoms and when they began

- medications they are taking

- sleep history

- location and any other specifics about pain

- jaw noises or abnormal jaw behaviors

- sleeping issues

- whether the patient is experiencing depression

The intake form helps me discuss issues with patients to help get a better understanding of their current situation, and it helps me target the source of their problem.

For instance, early in the health history discussion, I ask patients about pain, which is measured on a scale of zero to three, where zero is no pain, one is mild, two is moderate, and three is severe. The location of the pain is also very important, but it is not always an indicator of the actual source of the pain.

Sometimes, for example, when a person experiences pain in their neck, it's possible that their jaw is the cause. However, they'll usually go to their family doctor for a muscle relaxant or pain medication. When the pain returns, they'll go to their chiropractor—in fact, quite a few people who come to see me do so after having seen their chiropractor, often numerous times. One of my employees, Barbara, used to get a trigger point injection to relieve her back pain from her chiropractor once a month besides getting "adjustments" at least once a week. When my practice began evolving to treat TMJ, she recognized all of her symptoms as pointing to TMJ as a source. Now she wears a TMJ appliance and she hasn't been to the chiropractor since.

The health history also helps draw a picture of where a patient is in their care from other providers. For instance, when a person experiences pain for an extended time and is unable to find relief, they often end up depressed. They'll reach out to a physician to get a prescription for an antidepressant as a solution, only to have side effects that then must be addressed. Although it can be a sensitive issue with patients, by gaining their trust during the health history discussion, they will often share that kind of detail—again, information that needs to be known in order to reach an accurate diagnosis.

THE VISUAL AND PHYSICAL EXAMINATION

The health history discussion is followed by a visual examination of the teeth, the jaws, the nose, the tongue, the bite, and the muscles of the head and neck. These examinations look to target the source of the pain, determine whether there are any obstructions to airflow, and look at overall neurological connections.

The teeth. The start of the visual examination is a matter of simply looking inside the patient's mouth for abnormal wear or broken teeth. Teeth can break for a number of reasons—old fillings or hard foods, for instance—but a number of broken teeth, without any real reason, may be an indicator of TMJ and even a sleep disorder. These are signs of bruxism, or grinding and clenching. When I see bruxism, I start looking for other signs of a sleep disorder.

Gaps between teeth, for instance, could be a sign of a sleep disorder. I often get calls from restorative dentists, who are specialists in making teeth. They call me about patients who develop gaps between teeth after a crown has been placed on a tooth. I usually end up telling them the same thing: Send the patient for a sleep study, which usually determines the patient has sleep apnea. The gaps occur because the tongue is always moving around to create room for itself and to create an airway for the body as it struggles to breathe during sleep. Shifting teeth are common signs of a sleep disorder, and this can occur even after a person has braces.

Tongue thrust, or the tongue pushing its way forward in the mouth, can also create a gap or chronically open bite between the upper and lower teeth in the front of the mouth. With tongue thrust, the teeth are always gapped in the front, but they meet in the back, so there is more tendency to break the back teeth. I explain the mechanics of tongue thrust later in this chapter.

Abscesses or missing teeth may also indicate sleep apnea—the more missing teeth, the higher the chances of having sleep apnea.

The jaw bones and muscles. The examination also looks at the muscles of the face and jaws by palpating or pressing on these areas. The buccinators, or jaw muscles, can become very sore when a person grinds and clenches. I also check for pain or tenderness of the digastric muscles, which are below the chin.

Outside the mouth. The examination outside the mouth looks at the masseter muscles of the jaw, just beneath the cheek. When a person clenches and grinds excessively, they can change the shape of their face because the masseter muscle gets built up and becomes more prominent, making the face more angular.

Inside the mouth. I also look for tori, which are bony growths that can crowd the tongue and can be a symptom of clenching and grinding. Just as your other bones grow stronger when you work out, so do the bones inside your mouth. Tori are a good indicator of a teeth grinding or Bruxism, which could be a symptom of a sleep disorder. Tori can crowd the tongue and prevent it from being able to move forward inside the mouth, which causes it to move back into the airway.

The nose. An examination of the nose includes looking for polyps, inflammation, or other obstructions that may be causing a blockage. I want to see whether the patient could breathe better if they could get more air through their nose.

A visual exam of the nares (or the nostrils) looks for signs of a collapse. A collapse can make it difficult—or impossible—to breathe through the nose. Nasal valve collapse, as it's known, can be assessed by simply looking at the patient and having them take a deep breath.

Scans are also taken to look for sinus congestion. The scans are sent to an ENT for evaluation to see if, for instance, there is a deviated septum.

The examination of the head includes a look at the sinuses, eyes, and jaws to see whether they are fairly symmetrical and aligned.

The tongue and lips. Inside the mouth, I also look for tongue-tie. That occurs when the lingual frenulum is tight. The frenulum is the web-like tissue that attaches the tongue to the inside of the lower jaw behind the front teeth. When the mouth develops normally, the tongue plays an integral role in the development of the jaw and arch of the mouth, encouraging the jaw to grow outward and the arch to develop fully. Tongue-tie keeps the jaw from moving forward. It can also cause a speech impediment; unfortunately, some people go to speech therapy to help correct a problem that could be solved by a straightforward dental procedure that releases that frenulum, thereby releasing the tongue.

I also look for lip-tie, which is caused by the superior lingual frenulum, the web-like tissue between the upper lip and the gum in front of the upper teeth. Tongue-ties or lip-ties should be released at birth or in the infant stage.

The bite. Often when a person has TMJ, they find that opening their mouth wide causes considerable pain, so they stop opening their mouth fully. That's a mistake many people make because it can develop scar tissue and leads to diminished range of motion—the normal bite range is around 42 millimeters. One patient, Melissa, had been suffering from TMJ for twenty years and by the time she came to see me, she only had a bite range of 20 millimeters. She was just cutting her food up very small and sliding it in.

If you notice that your range of motion is smaller than it once was, seek treatment. At some point, treatment with an appliance will no longer be an option until a surgical cleaning (arthrocentesis) of the joint is performed.

Head, neck, and shoulder muscles. The physical exam also includes palpating or pressing on the muscles of the head, neck, and even the shoulders. Pain in these areas can indicate a sleep-disorder. That's because in the effort to open your airway, the body pushes the head forward on the shoulders. That causes pulling on the trapezius, which are the large muscles at the back of the neck and shoulders.

There are also muscles in the temple area, the temporalis, that can be affected by clenching and grinding.

After the visual exam, we then run a number of other tests to help arrive at the right diagnosis.

ADVANCED TESTING FOR TMJ

There are a number of advanced tests that are used to diagnose TMJ and sleep disorders. The testing used at my practice was developed by Drs. Steven Olmos and John Beck, an orthopedic surgeon. People often compensate for chronic pain for years, and often they seek out multiple solutions but never really get to the source of the problem. In their quest for answers, Olmos and Beck found that TMJ often caused pain in the head and other areas of the body, including the neck, shoulders, back, arms, and even the spine or the feet. That's why the tests we perform address so many other areas beyond just the temporomandibular joint, because the source of pain could be distant from the sight of pain.

Here are some of the more advanced tests used in diagnosing patients for TMJ and sleep disorders.

Photos to assess symmetry. Head shots—straight on and from the side—can assess whether a person has symmetry in the face, head, and neck. During a normal day's activities, asymmetry is not very noticeable because people are gesturing and moving around. But a photo can show whether a person tilts their head to one side, or whether it is in the forward position. When the head is forward, the back bends slightly, which can create neck problems.

Posture is a neurological process because muscles don't act without the brain telling them what to do. If the posture is off, then there are likely involuntary issues with the nervous system. Usually, a forward head position means a person is trying to breathe more easily.

Photos can help correlate what is suspected when X-rays, CT scans, and 3-D imaging tests are conducted.

X-rays, CT scans, and 3-D imaging with cone beam computed tomography (CBCT). X-rays, CT scans, and 3-D imaging reveal anatomic changes in the bones inside the mouth and in the jaw, head, and neck. Usually the results are read in the office and/or are sent to a radiologist for review.

The X-rays, CT scans, and 3-D images look at the condyle in the jaw, which, as I mentioned in Chapter 2, is the end portion of the jaw joint bone. The condyle should fit neatly into the center of the fossa, which is the concave, bowl-like area in the skull. If the images show the condyle to be positioned in front or back of the fossa, then we know that it is displaced.

The images are done using cone beam computed tomography (CBCT), a type of X-ray in which the rays during the scanning procedure form a cone. The cone gives a more comprehensive view of the structures of the areas scanned—roughly everything from the neck up.

When reviewing the 3-D images, I look for anything that seems out of the ordinary. For instance, with one patient, I found what was ultimately diagnosed by a radiologist as carotid artery calcification, or blockage of arteries that indicate the patient is in danger of having a stroke.

The 3-D scan also has special software that lets us see the volume of the airway. The display is color-coded, with different colors indicating the amount of airflow. Black means very little air is getting through.

Joint vibration analysis (JVA). A JVA is a noninvasive test in which the patient wears a headset that records the vibration in the jaw during movement. It can reveal whether the joint is experiencing inflammation, is essentially immobile, or is bone on bone. The JVA can determine the degree of degradation in the tissue between the condyle and fossa bones (of the jaw) and the masseter muscle (in the cheek).

Motor nerve reflex testing. When photos, X-rays, CT scans, and/or 3-D imaging reveal issues with the nervous system, then the reflexes are tested. The motor nerve reflex test is an orthopedic neurological test, developed by Drs. Olmos and Beck, which looks specifically for sources of pain.

When a bite is misaligned, it can affect the muscles and nerves throughout the body, causing spasms not only in your face, jaw, neck, and shoulders, but also pinching the nerves in your arms. When that happens, a person can experience numbness, tingling, or a prickling sensation in the arms, fingers, and hands. Some people even report that their grip strength is lessened.

The **light/dark motor nerve reflex test** involves the patient looking straight ahead at a neutrally colored wall, then holding their arms up so their pinkies are parallel to the floor. I then push their arms together and ask them to resist, which they usually can. Then I have them close their eyes and I push their arms together again. If they can't resist my push with one or both arms, then I know there is dystrophy (tissue degeneration) somewhere in their nervous system. The same happens with the **scratch test**; instead of pushing on the arms, I lightly scratch the nerve in the arms and then push their arms down.

One patient, Elise, had been in pain for about a month and had lost about ten pounds during that time. She was already diagnosed with myasthenia gravis, a neuromuscular disease that causes muscle weakness. When I tested her reflexes, in spite of her weakness, she was able to resist when I pushed on her arm. That led me to determine that she did not have a TMJ problem. In an effort to get to the source of her pain, I dug deeper into her history and found that, because of her disease, she had poor balance and had suffered a serious fall that knocked out two of her teeth. A dentist had managed to put the teeth back in, but they were positioned to where they were pushed back a little, which was different than before the fall—Elise had pictures that supported my assessment. I examined her mouth further and found that the placement of the two teeth wasn't permitting her bite to meet in the back. I sent her to an orthodontist who was able to, over time, reposition her teeth to their previous position, eliminating Elise's need for any sort of appliance. As my mentor, Dr. Olmos, always says: "There is no minimum daily requirement for plastic in the mouth." In other words, getting to the source in cases like Elise's can eliminate the need for an appliance and determine the appropriate care.

Similar to the light/dark and scratch tests, the **posture test** looks for dystrophy in the nervous system. This test involves the patient standing against a wall to check for posture and balance. Against the wall, a person's center of gravity is over their feet and they tend to be more stable; away from the wall, a slight push can off-balance them.

Magnetic Resonance Imaging (MRI). In some cases, I have the patient undergo an MRI to determine whether the disc in the jaw is in place or is misaligned. An MRI is more common if there has been a trauma to the face, such as in a car accident. However, this test is less commonly used because it is an additional expense, and the diagnosis for TMJ can usually be made through other testing.

INITIAL SIGNS OF A SLEEP-DISORDER

When I suspect a sleep disorder, I begin asking questions, such as whether the patient tosses and turns at night. Often, I find, children are better at answering this question than adults are. Usually I'll ask something like: "When you wake up, are your covers off the bed? Are your sheets all messed up? Is your head on the other side of the bed than when you went to sleep?" If the patient tells me they wake up in a completely different position and that their bedsheets are in complete disarray, I know they likely have some sort of sleep disorder. When you're in deep sleep, you shouldn't be tossing and turning.

Here are some other symptoms that may indicate a sleep disorder:

Snoring. Snoring is the classic symptom that a person may have sleep-disordered breathing or sleep apnea. Even if someone claims they have a "dainty" snore, it's still a snore. More often, patients seek help because someone else—even someone sleeping in another room—has told them they snore to the point that it is disturbing their sleep; I call that "secondary snore," which affects the sleep of the non-snorer.

Tongue position. The position of the tongue may indicate a sleep disorder. A tongue that sits in the back of the throat is more likely to be an obstruction than one that rests in the lower cavity of the mouth, behind the teeth. The more space the tongue occupies in the mouth, the greater your chances of having a sleep disorder. A tongue that rests in the back of the airway is a dangerous thing: it can literally kill you because it blocks the airway.

A tongue with a coating can also be an indicator of a sleep disorder since it may indicate chronic mouth breathing, which can occur with sleep-disordered breathing or sleep apnea. Mouth breathing dries out the tongue, which leads to a coating on it.

A tongue with scalloped edges may also indicate a sleep disorder. Scalloping can occur when a person has a very narrow lower jaw, and there is not enough room for the tongue, causing it to curl up, or scallop, along either side.

Tongue thrust, which I discussed earlier, is a key symptom of a sleep disorder. The tongue is the strongest muscle in the body, and when it is working to help you breathe at night, it can apply up to 500 grams of pressure to the front teeth. Every time you swallow, you use your tongue, which happens about two thousand times a day. If it pushes forward out of a desire to help open your airway, then it is moving between your upper and lower teeth two thousand times a day—that's how it creates the gaps and chronically open bite I discussed earlier.

Some people are fitted for braces two or three times because they have an open bite, a space between their upper and lower teeth that just won't close. That's because they have a sleep problem, not an orthodontic problem.

The airway (nose to throat). Blockage of the airway can occur in the nose or by the tongue, which I've already discussed. Tonsils, especially in young people, can constrict the airway. The uvula can also block the airway if it is oversized. An exam of the airway also involves looking at the soft palate, which is the area on the roof of the mouth that slopes back into the throat. A loose or drooping soft palate can also block the airway.

The teeth. As with TMJ, the condition of the teeth can be an indicator of a sleep disorder. Symptoms with the teeth that I look for include the number of missing teeth; a narrow arch, which can crowd the tongue; crooked teeth, from the tongue moving around trying to open the airway; and broken teeth and crowns, which occur when a person grinds their teeth at night.

Neck size. As I mentioned in the last chapter, neck size is another potential indicator of sleep-disordered breathing or sleep apnea. A neck size greater than 17 inches on a man and greater than 16 inches on a woman may be an indicator of a sleep disorder.

ADVANCED TESTING FOR SLEEP DISORDERED BREATHING

Sleep apnea must be diagnosed by a medical doctor who specializes in sleep disorders. That diagnosis can only be made after the patient has undergone a polysomnography (PSG), or sleep study.

Before sending someone out to have a sleep study, we have them complete the Epworth Sleepiness Scale (ESS), a short questionnaire developed by Dr. Murray Johns of Melbourne, Australia. The ESS is used to measure a person's likelihood of dozing off in specific situations. The score from the ESS determines whether a person has daytime sleepiness ranging from "normal lower" to "severe excessive."

There is also a version of the scale for youth, The Epworth Sleepiness Scale for Children and Adolescents (ESS-CHAD), that lets us see whether a young person has a sleep disorder.

The Sleep Study

There are two types of sleep studies today—one conducted in a sleep lab and the other, a take-home version.

During the sleep study conducted in a lab, monitors are attached to the patient and technicians watch the person sleep from another room. The leads are attached to the head, nose, fingertips, and other areas on the body.

Because sleep studies conducted in a lab are considerably more expensive, and insurance does not always pay for the test, many people opt for a take-home version. The take-home version is typically self-pay, but it costs less. The take-home versions are not as sensitive, and therefore not always as accurate as the test done in the sleep clinic: sometimes the take-home test must be taken more than once to get an accurate reading, it may miss a diagnosis of mild sleep apnea altogether, or it may misreport the severity of sleep apnea.

The study measures what is known as the Apnea-Hypopnea Index (AHI) along with oxygen levels in the bloodstream. The index is the average of the number of apnea (pauses in breathing) and hypopnea (abnormally shallow or low levels of breathing) events that occur during the period measured. The sleep study also checks for oxygen levels. Optimal oxygen level in the blood is 90 percent.

The resulting AHI of a sleep study indicate the severity of the sleep apnea:

- 0 to 4.9 is normal

- 5 to 15 is mild

- 16 to 30 is moderate

- Over 30 is severe

When the sleep study reveals an average in the 0 to 4.9 range, then snoring is typically the only issue addressed, and that can be done with an oral appliance. The American Academy of Sleep Medicine recognizes that mild and even moderate sleep apnea can be treated with oral appliances. Severe sleep apnea, however, is typically addressed with a CPAP machine.

If a person has a diagnosis of TMJ, I inform the sleep clinic prior to the sleep study so the doctor is aware that the patient will need combination treatment, which will depend in part on the severity of their sleep apnea. For instance, a person with severe sleep apnea may need a CPAP machine, but they may also need an appliance to treat their TMJ.

Since appliances tend to be easier to tolerate than CPAPs, people usually use them more often—they are more compliant than using the machine. Let's look at these treatment options, as well as others.

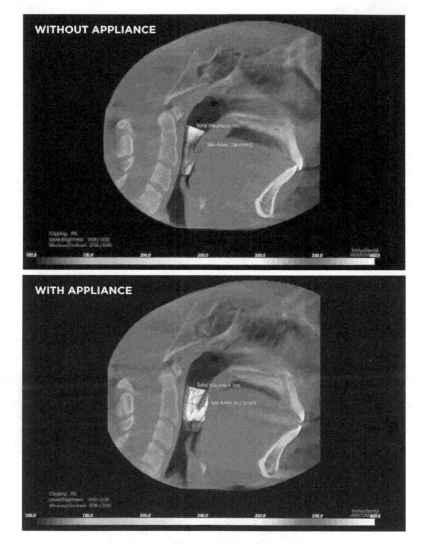

AHI without appliance: 13.5, AHI with appliance: 3.0

CHAPTER 4

DIFFERENT TREATMENTS FOR DIFFERENT PATIENTS

"The things that make me different are the things that make me."

—WINNIE THE POOH

Bart came to see me at age fifty for problems with his TMJ. Thirty years earlier, he had undergone a procedure known as arthrocentesis, which is when sterile saline is injected into the jaw joint to clean it out and loosen it up. At the time, he was told that he would probably need the procedure again later in life, and it appeared that day had arrived.

When he came in for his appointment, the right side of his face—the side with the TMJ pain—was swollen and his jaw was locked to the point that he was unable to sufficiently open his mouth. To get relief, he had been to see his dentist, who referred him to the TMJ & Sleep Therapy Centre of North Texas.

Since the arthrocentesis was really a last-resort option, I gave him some anti-inflammatory medication, muscle relaxants, and cold laser treatment to reduce the inflammation. By reducing the inflammation in his jaw, we were able to help him open his mouth wider. Then I fashioned a temporary appliance for him to use at night to prevent him from clenching and grinding while he waited on his permanent appliance. This relieved Bart's situation, and in the end, he didn't need arthrocentesis.

In the past, a traditional night guard was considered to be the best solution for TMJ symptoms. However, that may actually worsen the problem, since it can take up space in the mouth that is needed for the tongue—and which may already be lacking. That, as you have read in the previous chapters, can lead to a sleep disorder.

In my practice, appliance therapy addresses the anatomical problem that causes TMJ, helping to open the jaw slightly and preventing clenching and grinding.

When it comes to the temporomandibular joint, it's preferable to try conservative treatments first because one of the pitfalls of surgery for TMJ is the scar tissue that develops afterward. In the most severe cases—those where the patient undergoes multiple surgeries—the scar tissue itself may eventually require surgery all its own. Even after surgery, in most cases, the patient must still wear an appliance to help prevent that buildup of scar tissue.

When conservative treatment is insufficient, surgery may be the best answer for TMJ. However, surgery of the TMJ for the management of chronic pain has a history of unpredictable results. Common reasons for failure of TMJ surgery include:

Failure to eliminate the cause of the problem, besides the obvious pathology. Unless the cause of the TMJ is addressed, there is a higher chance of recurrence of the condition. In many cases, for instance, the cause of bruxism is an obstructed nasal airway. Even other discomforts on the body—pain in a foot or lower back, for instance—can cause a person to grind their teeth at night. That's why it's crucial to look for the true source of the pain before treating for TMJ (or for a sleep disorder). For instance, Joshua, a patient of mine, was diagnosed and being treated for sleep apnea but was still grinding his teeth because he was still constantly waking at night. Finally, he revealed that he had pain in his hip and was putting off surgery. I had him apply lidocaine cream to his hip at bedtime, and he was able to sleep through the night. In his case, the pain in his hip was disturbing his sleep, causing him to clench and grind his teeth. He's a perfect example of how "every TMJ patient is ten patients in one," and how getting to the source of the problem is like peeling back an onion, one layer at a time.

Testing them may show they also have pain in their foot or in their neck. As each of the patient's chief complaints is addressed one at a time, other complaints rise to the forefront. For example, when Dr. Olmos addressed my TMJ pain, my neck was still hurting. So he tested me again and found the problems with my feet. Once those problems were addressed, then my jaw pain went away. During all the testing, he discovered that I might have sleep-disordered breathing, so I went for a sleep study and, sure enough, I tested as having moderate sleep apnea. After peeling back all my layers, one at a time, and addressing each individual issue, I no longer have pain.

Incorrect diagnosis. Myofascial pain disorder and TMJ disorder have similar symptoms, making them difficult to accurately diagnose. Myofascial pain involves the facial muscles, while TMJ can involve the joint and surrounding tissue. An incorrect diagnosis can lead to inappropriate treatment with surgery, when medical management would resolve the problems.

CURRENT SURGICAL PROCEDURES FOR TMJ

When the patient really has no other choice because of function, pain, or the fact that conservative efforts have failed, then there are some more aggressive treatments and surgical options that may be considered. Note that even when surgery is the only option left, the best outcomes are those where the patient participates in proper postoperative care and rehabilitation.

Aggressive treatments and surgical interventions for severe TMJ include:

Arthrocentesis and arthroscopy. These are minimally invasive surgical techniques that involve joint lavage, which essentially means washing, cleaning, or rinsing out the joint. These procedures can be used for a joint that is locked shut, causes chronic pain, or has hypomobility (decreased movement). Arthrocentesis is frequently used to treat a jaw with painful, limited range of motion.

Injections. Injections of corticosteroids into the joint may be helpful in relieving pain and improving mobility.

Modified condylotomy. This is a surgical procedure performed on the mandible (jawbone), but not in the joint itself. It can be helpful for treating pain when conservative treatments fail to do so. The surgery involves removing part of the condyle to allow better range of movement. In some cases, patients can get good results with an appliance instead of this procedure; the appliance allows the inflammation to subside and the joint to reshape.

Total joint replacement. In the following situations, a total joint replacement may be the best solution for TMJ:

- Condylar resorption—one or both mandibular condyles (balls) are broken down because of bone resorption.

- Arthritis—including osteoarthritis or rheumatoid arthritis, in which the disc is worn down and there is bone-on-bone grating.

- Ankylosis—a jaw locked for a long time develops scar tissue to the point that the joints are beginning to fuse together, creating stiffness and restricting movement; the only way to release the jaw is through a surgical procedure.

- Congenital deformation or absence of the TMJ—a malformed or damaged joint on one side of the face can cause TMJ on the other side; these can worsen with facial development, so should be addressed when occurring in youth.

- Trauma—can come from internal forces, such as grinding of teeth, or from external forces, such as a fractured condyle resulting from a car accident or work-related incident.

CURRENT SURGICAL PROCEDURES
FOR SLEEP DISORDERS

Like TMJ surgical procedures, there are surgical options for sleep-disordered breathing and sleep apnea. Again, conservative treatments should be tried before many of these options.

Nasal valves. As I mentioned in Chapter 2, the nasal passages are the beginning of the airway. Nasal passages that are collapsed partially or completely make it difficult to breathe. Surgery to correct the problem includes rebuilding the structures of the nose to open the airways and give the nose more stability. When I identify a patient with nasal valve obstruction, I refer them to an ENT for a possible Spira Latera procedure.

Hypertrophied turbinates. Turbinates are the structures inside the nose that help to regulate airflow. When these become hypertrophied (enlarged) by allergies, chronic inflammation, or other irritants in the environment, they can become an obstruction in the airway. Surgical treatment options include fracturing the structure to open the airway, removing a portion of bone, cauterizing the tissue, using radiofrequency to shrink the tissue, or excising the tissue.

A deviated septum can also obstruct the nasal passage. A true deviation is only diagnosed using X-ray. Treatment these days is a simple procedure that is mildly painful and allows the patient to return to work the following day.

Uvulopalatopharyngoplasty (UPPP). This is a somewhat drastic surgical procedure that involves partial removal of the uvula and reducing the edges of the soft palate. UPPP is a permanent procedure that is not always successful. Complications of UPPP include pain and swelling, bleeding, risk of infection, problems with swallowing, and a loss of taste.

Macroglossia reduction. For patients with a large tongue, one that crowds the space inside the mouth, there is a procedure known as macroglossia (tongue) reduction, which physically reduces the size of the tongue. Few people actually have a tongue that is too large. Most of the time, the problem is narrow arches, which can be corrected with orthodontics using expanders.

Tonsils and adenoid removal. As I mentioned previously, especially in children, removal of the tonsils and adenoids is a fairly common surgical intervention for airway obstruction.

Orthognathic surgery. This surgery involves actually breaking the jaw (upper, lower, or both), and then bringing the jaw(s) and tongue forward to increase the airway space at the back of the throat. Although it's a fairly drastic surgical procedure—and costly, generally around $50,000—it has a greater than 90 percent success rate. Patients who undergo this surgery are usually also fitted with braces.

Hyoid bone. Rarely is moving the hyoid bone an option for TMJ, however it is considered in some cases. The hyoid is a bone in the neck that can be moved, bringing along with it many muscles that are attached to the tongue. When the hyoid bone is lowered, it stretches the tongue out and opens the airway.

Hypoglossal nerve stimulation. The hypoglossal nerve supplies the muscles to the tongue. When the nerve is stimulated, it causes the tongue to move forward and out of the airway. Basically, the treatment involves giving your tongue periodic, minor shocks throughout the night; reportedly, the treatment works pretty well once the patient gets accustomed to the periodic shocks.

Genioglossus advancement. The genioglossus is a muscle in the tongue. Genioglossus advancement is a surgical procedure that involves moving the anchor for the tongue (inside the lower jaw) forward to create more space in the airway.

Maxillomandibular advancement (MMA). Also known as bimaxillary advancement (Bi-Max), or maxillomandibular osteotomy (MMO), moves the maxilla (upper jaw) and the mandible (lower jaw) forward. Although the success rate is good with MMA, the recovery time is fairly long considering that the facial structure is changed and must heal in its new position.

As you can see, there are a number of surgical options for TMJ and sleep apnea. However, as I mentioned, I recommend trying non-surgical options first, for a number of reasons. Surgery is permanent, and not always successful. In fact, with many of the aforementioned procedures, the success rate is pretty low.

With intraoral appliances becoming more advanced, many of these surgeries are being performed less often. Oral appliances are far easier on the patient than surgery, and they have a better success rate—depending on patient compliance. People with TMJ are often used to using a night guard or retainer, so getting used to an intraoral appliance is a fairly easy transition.

The American Academy of Sleep Medicine recommends that patients with mild and even moderate sleep apnea start out with intraoral appliances. For more serious cases of sleep apnea, a CPAP is recommended. However, when compliance becomes an issue, then oral appliances are also a viable companion option for sleep apnea sufferers. Oral appliances are portable, they let you sleep in any position, and they don't disturb sleeping partners (like a CPAP machine often does). Only when oral appliances and/or CPAP machines don't work should surgery be considered.

CUSTOMIZED TREATMENT

Treating patients is about more than just giving them an appliance, it's about looking at many different components of their health. At TMJ & Sleep Therapy Centre of North Texas, we look at the whole person in order to get to the source of the problem and provide the right treatment. When that treatment involves oral appliances, there are several to choose from. Here are some of the treatments and appliances prescribed for patients dealing with TMJ and/or a sleep disorder.

Exercises. Breathing through the nose is the most important thing you can do for your health. Some exercises can help train the upper lip to stay down, allowing for breathing more consistently through the nose. A mouth that is open too much can result in passive inhalation of air, which can cause the nose to essentially stop working.

Exercises include the Buteyko Method, which involves breath holding, nasal breathing, and relaxation. Another exercise involves taking a breath, holding the nose closed, pacing until a breath is needed, and then only breathing through the nose.

DR. KRISH'S TIPS FOR A GOOD NIGHT'S SLEEP

Lack of sleep can leave you fatigued and with a weakened immune system, making you more susceptible to infections. It can also decrease your mental acuity, disrupt natural hormone levels, and lead to a variety of other, significant health problems. Here are some tips to help you get some quality shut-eye!

1. **Set your clock:** Set an alarm thirty minutes before you want to go to bed so that you can remind yourself to shut off electronic devices and start to unwind. Go to bed at the same time every night.

2. **Skip that afternoon pick-me-up:** Limit caffeine intake about six hours before bedtime. Also limit alcoholic drinks to no more than two in a sitting.

3. **Set the mood:** Your bedroom should be an oasis; you should have dark shades covering all windows, no noise, and the temperature should be set between 68° and 72°F.

4. **Do not disturb:** Flashing screens and the light on cell phones and iPads stimulate our brains and make it difficult to relax. Ideally, you should step away from tech two hours before bedtime. At the very least, turn on "Night Shift" if your phone has

that capability and when you do put your phone down, set it for "Do Not Disturb."

5.   **Ritual:** Set bedtime rituals. Warm baths, listening to relaxing music, and reading before bed are just a few examples. Getting into a nightly routine will signify to your brain when it's time to start relaxing and preparing for sleep.

6.   **No midnight snack:** Eat dinner about three to four hours before bedtime. This will give your body a chance to digest your food and be able to fully relax.

7.   **Use your bed only as a bed:** Doing work or other stressful activities while in bed can make it difficult for your brain to relax when it's time to sleep. Go into a different room or least off your bed so that when your body hits the mattress, your brain knows it can start to relax.

8.   **Get moving:** Exercising on a regular basis is not only good for your body and overall health but also for your sleep! A solid thirty minutes of daily exercise can make a huge difference in quality of sleep.

9.   **Naptime?:** Skip that afternoon catnap. Napping during the day can make it difficult to fall asleep at night, making you more tired the next day... it's a never-ending cycle! If you really feel like you need to recharge, don't nap for longer than twenty minutes.

10. **Rule Out a Sleep Disorder:** Trouble falling asleep, waking up regularly during the night, and snoring are just a few indicators that you might have a sleep disorder. Waking up not feeling refreshed is not natural and might be an indicator of a more serious problem. Dr. Krish's comprehensive exam can help get to the source of your sleep problems.

Anti-inflammatories. When the nasal passages are blocked by inflammation, over-the-counter sprays may help. Steroids may also be prescribed on a short-term basis only, typically two weeks.

Commonly prescribed medications for orofacial and TMJ pain include nonsteroidal, anti-inflammatory drugs (NSAIDs).

Natural muscle relaxants can reduce muscle spasms and relax tight muscles. These are typically short-term solutions used until treatment takes effect. These include:

- Chamomile, magnesium, cherry juice, cayenne pepper.

- Magnesium, which is found in bananas, almonds, and legumes.

- Chamomile tea or oil can also be used to massage sore muscles. The anti-inflammatory antioxidant properties can help relax muscles naturally.

Botox also blocks muscle contractions and is given for temporary relief; however, it does not address the cause of the muscle spasm. Only appliances will actually correct the problem by correcting the cranial position of the jaw.

Cold laser. For patients who are in great pain or have a locked jaw (open or closed), we use a cold laser therapy before treating with an appliance. The cold laser reduces inflammation, which helps relieve pain and loosens the jaw.

Patients with locked jaw must be treated right away, otherwise scar tissue can develop in the joint. I had one patient who had been locked for twenty years. When I asked her how she ate, she said she just cut everything up into small pieces. After twenty years of being locked, she needed surgery to undo the damage. But most patients can find relief for a locked jaw with cold laser, muscle relaxers, nitrous oxide, or other nonsurgical options.

Cold laser also works to loosen the neck and shoulder muscles when someone's posture has been affected—that head-forward position I discussed—by poor breathing and they are putting extra weight on their neck and shoulders. Cold laser can loosen the muscles, allowing us to get a proper bite for creating appliances.

Appliances. There are many appliances available, each with their own benefits and features. Most are designed to decompress the joint and help reduce inflammation there. At TMJ & Sleep Therapy Centre of North Texas, we use different appliances for different situations.

A decompression appliance is for people who are grinding their teeth at night, but the source of their pain is undetermined. This appliance controls parafunctional activity, such as clenching and grinding, and reduces inflammation.

A TMJ-only appliance keeps the lower jaw forward. This is one of the appliances we use most often. This appliance reduces inflammation, prevents locking in the supine position, and reduces forces of clenching and grinding.

Daytime-only appliances are worn during the daytime for patients to continue healing a jaw joint for twenty-four hours a day by keeping it stable, which helps reduce inflammation. Most patients are successfully weaned off these after wearing them for ten to twelve weeks.

Performance (sport) appliances are used by many athletes. I created one for my daughter, Brittany, and she reported that she was able to run longer without getting tired because she could breathe easier when wearing the appliance. These are custom-made appliances that are worn during exercise and help position the jaw to open the airway.

Three-appliance therapy. At TMJ & Sleep Therapy Centre of North Texas, we have a three-appliance therapy designed to move the joint and surrounding muscles. The therapy consists of a night appliance that is actually two appliances—upper and lower—that keep the teeth apart to prevent grinding. Since the goal of the therapy is to heal the joint, we need that joint to be as stable as possible. That's where the third appliance—a daytime appliance mentioned earlier—comes in. The daytime appliance keeps the joint stable, helping to reduce inflammation and allowing healing to continue nearly uninterrupted. The daytime appliance is worn for ten to twelve weeks, at which time the patient is weaned off it. After that, for most patients, only the night appliances are worn going forward.

For about 10 percent of patients, relief comes from a second phase of treatment, which involves orthodontics customized to the patient's needs. For instance, crowns on the back teeth can help retain a vertical dimension in the mouth, which is key to healing. Or, in the case of one school vice principal, a daytime appliance made of material that looks like real teeth proved to be the best solution after other treatments, including chiropractic and injections, ultimately no longer provided relief.

Treatment with the three-appliance therapy usually lasts three months. Relief can be felt within two weeks of wearing the devices for some patients but takes a little longer for others. The nighttime appliance must be worn long-term for a lifetime of relief. The only way to avoid wearing the nighttime appliance is to correct the teeth, bite, and airway with functional orthodontics (braces) that take into account the airway.

These days, models of the patient's teeth—which are used to create the appliances—are computerized. Fitting is also done using phonetics to help capture a 3-D picture of the position when the jaw is forward and open enough to correct the problem. The appliance gets rid of cants in the mouth, leveling everything off to where it is parallel to the ground.

CPAP AND ORAL APPLIANCES FOR SLEEP APNEA

CPAP is a common—and often necessary—treatment for sleep apnea. CPAP (continuous positive airway pressure) is a machine that pumps air through a hose connected to a mask that is worn at night by a person suffering from obstructive sleep apnea (OSA). It helps an OSA sufferer breathe more easily during sleep. However, many people prefer to try other treatments because CPAP is cumbersome and can cause dry mouth since it blows air down the wearer's throat. These and other unwelcome features lead some people to avoid using their CPAP machine nightly as prescribed.

Appliances are especially useful for patients who have difficulty with CPAP machines. Today, some patients opt for hybrid therapy involving both an appliance and a CPAP, which means a greater chance of success with treatment, and a greater chance of compliance. With hybrid therapy, the CPAP wearer only needs a nasal cannula, which pumps air through the nose only. No need for the full mask to be worn at night. Hybrid therapy also allows for lower-pressure air to be pumped to the wearer, since the appliance is doing some of the work of opening the airway.

THE GOOD NEWS

With TMJ disorder, the joint deteriorates. But the good news is that the affected joint can remodel itself once the inflammation has been controlled.

Unlike other joints in the body, the TMJ is structured in a way that is a little different. What makes the TMJ different from other joints? The articulating surfaces, or moving surfaces, are covered with fibrocartilage, which is cartilage that contains collagen fibers. Other joints in the body are hyaline cartilage, which is a translucent substance. Fibrocartilage is more durable than hyaline cartilage and therefore less likely to be damaged by the effects of aging and breakdown over the years.

The results of experimental animal work have shown the mandibular condylar cartilage, which is part of the TMJ, is capable of regeneration after injury. That's what preserves the jawbone after an injury.[20]

Currently, there is no cure for TMJ, but with treatment and therapy, there is relief. TMJ and sleep disorders cannot be fixed with medication. The causes are typically structural, involving cranial development. Most of the damage happens at night, when your body is unconscious and cannot control its movements. That's why it's necessary to wear appliances for life to correct the position of the face and jaws. That is, unless the issues are addressed during the developmental stages—in childhood.

---

20   P. D. Robinson, "Articular Cartilage of the Temporomandibular Joint: Can It Regenerate," *Annals of the Royal College of Surgeons of England* 75, no. 4 (1993): 231–36.

In the next chapter, I'll discuss how problems begin and what can be done in the early stages of life to reduce or eliminate disorders later.

CHAPTER 5

YOUTH SNORING—IT'S A PROBLEM, IT'S NOT "CUTE"

"Laugh and the world laughs with you, snore and you sleep alone."

—ANTHONY BURGESS

Amy was twenty years old when she came to see me for help resolving her facial pain and sleeping problems. At the time, she had already been on antidepressants since she was fourteen years old. The medications she took during the day kept her awake at night, so she had to take other medications to help her sleep at night. These medications also made her clench and grind her teeth.

We treated her for TMJ with appliance therapy and at her six-month follow-up appointment, she told us she was no longer on any medications.

It's a common story—youth (and adults) are put on medications, or they take over-the-counter medications, when the problem is related to a structural issue that can be corrected with therapy, or it's related to sleep. When a child wakes up with a headache, he or she is often given a dose of ibuprofen or acetaminophen. When they have trouble breathing through their nose, they are often diagnosed with asthma or chronic allergies, for which they are prescribed an antihistamine or a steroid. Steroids, by the way, are typically used only for a short time to control pain and other symptoms. Long-term use of steroids has many negative side effects.

IT'S ALL ABOUT SLEEP AND BREATHING

Sleep problems often start in childhood yet go undetected because parents sometimes don't realize there is a problem, and teachers and coaches only see a problem child. No one is relating the child's problems to sleep. When adults have sleep problems, they can drink coffee to stay awake, but kids don't have similar solutions for staying awake. So their problems manifest in hyperactivity, poor school performance, and bad behavior at home and at school.

But there are signs and symptoms that shouldn't be ignored when it comes to children and sleep disordered breathing.

SYMPTOMS OF SLEEP DISORDERED BREATHING IN CHILDREN INCLUDE:

- Snoring
- Daytime sleepiness
- Daytime crankiness
- Disheveled bedding
- Difficulty waking
- Malformed teeth
- Bedwetting
- ADD/ADHD
- Frequent infections

- Fidgeting

- Easily stimulated or distracted

As in adults, snoring is a primary indicator of sleep-disordered breathing or sleep apnea in a child. People often see a small child asleep and emitting a tiny snore. "That's so cute," they say, ignoring that it's potentially a sign the baby is not getting enough air. Now, every child who snores does not necessarily have sleep apnea. According to Gary Freed, DO, professor of pediatrics and director of the Pediatric Sleep Laboratory at Emory University School of Medicine in Atlanta, while 7 to 12 percent of children snore, only 1 to 3 percent of children who snore have sleep apnea.[21] Still, snoring should never be ignored, because it could be the first sign of a much larger problem.

Daytime sleepiness or crankiness is another big indicator of a sleep disorder. Often, children are misdiagnosed as having ADD, ADHD, or other behavioral problems that disrupt their school performance and daily lives. They're categorized as "problem children" because they are so disruptive in school. But the truth is, all they're trying to do is stay awake. Lack of sleep can even lead to aggressive behavior, such as bullying.[22]

Disheveled bedding is another sign of a sleep disorder. Parents may chalk up a messy bed as just the way their child is. And, as I mentioned in Chapter 3, sometimes children are a better judge of their sleeping problems than are their parents. Their parents may think their child sleeps just fine; they may say their child doesn't need a sleep study. But the child will tell me their bed is a mess when they wake up, or they'll tell me straight-out: "I can't sleep."

---

21 "Sleep apnea in school-age kids," DIYhealthacademy, https://diyhealthacademy. com/sleep-apnea-in-school-age-kids/.

22 Walker, *Why We Sleep*.

A child who constantly fidgets, who is easily stimulated or easily distracted, has some of the malformed teeth problems that I've discussed in previous chapters, or has night terrors may also be suffering from a sleep disorder.

Take Cheyenne, for instance. At age five, she already had tongue thrust from sucking her thumb at night. Cayenne pepper on her thumb didn't resolve the problem because she loved hot foods. She would just lick the pepper off and then keep right on sucking. When her mother brought Cheyenne to my office, I came up with a solution that actually worked: I taped a straw to her thumb as if it were a splint, wrapping the tape around her wrist to keep it secure. Sure enough, in two days, she was cured of thumb-sucking.

But Cheyenne also had night terrors and would wake up screaming and would tell her mother she thought she was going to die. I had her go for a sleep study, which revealed that she had sleep apnea. I fitted her with an appliance, which helped her breathe better, sleep through the night, and wake more rested in the morning. It also solved her night terrors, which were due to her inability to breathe properly.

Another symptom of a sleep problem in children is frequent infections, which are caused by mouth breathing. It's crucial for children—and adults—to breathe through the nose, whether asleep or awake. The nose is designed to capture bacteria, dust, and other airborne particles before they can reach the lungs. It is also designed to warm the air we breathe, reducing constriction of the bronchioles, which are vital for air distribution in the lungs. And air breathed through the nose mixes with nitric oxide produced by the sinuses, which is a natural antioxidant for the entire body.

A baby should sleep with its mouth closed. But the brain doesn't care whether air gets in through the nose or the mouth; it only cares about making sure the person stays alive. If a baby is sleeping with their mouth open, it means their nose has stopped working. Now, a stuffy nose from a cold is one thing; when a child (or adult) has a cold, they tend to breathe through their mouth. However, if their nose can be cleared, then everything else will take care of itself. If, instead, the child continues breathing through the mouth, then the tonsils, which act like big lymph nodes trying to protect the body, become enlarged. That can lead to a blockage of the airway.

Multiple ear infections can be a sign that a baby is not breathing right because a clogged nose can ultimately infect the ear. All-natural drops can shrink the tissues inside the nose, making it easier to breathe.

The need for ear tubes can also be a breathing/sleep disorder indicator. Ear tubes are usually needed because the Eustachian tubes in babies are very small and very close to the mouth. When a child whose jaw has not developed downward tries to swallow, anything they're trying to swallow (milk, water, etc.) ends up draining into the Eustachian tube. That's the reason it is important to position the baby correctly during feeding. You know how hard it is to lie down and try to drink through a straw? Well, it's no easier for a baby to try to drink from a bottle while lying down with their head on a couple of pillows. In order to keep from drowning, the child will push their tongue forward to control how much fluid goes down their throat. Where does the rest of the fluid go? It goes up into the ears, which can lead to infections. Chronic nasal obstruction is a common symptom of allergic rhinitis (hay fever). Since the nasal airway is the normal route for breathing, nasal congestion can cause snoring and sleep apnea.

PROBLEMS NOW LEAD TO PROBLEMS LATER

The problem with ignoring the signs and symptoms of a sleep disorder in a child is that early developmental problems can lead to problems later in life. Jay is a perfect example of that.

Jay was a sixteen-year-old who was getting ready to go to camp for the summer. While he was looking forward to going away to camp, he was anxious because, at night, he couldn't control his bladder. At his age, he was still wetting the bed. Originally, I recommended that he undergo a sleep study. But he and his mom told me that he didn't have trouble sleeping, the problem was that he slept so deeply he did not wake to go the bathroom when he needed to. However, it's not common for a young person to have to get out of bed in the middle of the night to go to the bathroom. That's something that happens more commonly as a person ages.

Finally, Jay agreed to the sleep study, which—sure enough—found that he had sleep apnea. The solution for the problem was fairly simple. I fitted him with an intraoral appliance that he wore at night to help with his breathing.

At first, he didn't want to wear the appliance, believing it couldn't possibly solve his problem. But it wasn't long before he was no longer wetting the bed. In fact, his behavior was better in school and he even saw an improvement in his grades.

Even children and teens need help addressing their TMJ and sleep disorders. That's my goal, to eliminate those health issues early so that children can lead productive, pain-free, label-free, medication-free lives.

TMJ and sleep disorders are problems that start at an early age, as I'll explain in the next chapter.

CHAPTER 6

PREVENTION—STRUCTURAL/FUNCTIONAL ISSUES IN EARLY LIFE

"An once of prevention is worth a pound of cure."

—HENRY DE BRACTON

One day I was talking to ten-year-old Elena's mother, who casually shared with me that her daughter was using anti-wrinkle cream for dark shadows under her eyes. I hadn't really seen Elena for a while, but when she came into the room I saw right away that her lower jaw was very retruded or set further back on her face. She had a bad thumb-sucking habit that was beginning to cause a gap in her teeth, which would ultimately give her a triangular arch and buck teeth. Without addressing the issue, she was also in danger of stunting the growth of her lower front teeth. Elena was scheduled to begin orthodontic treatment in a few months, but I told her mother that I thought there might be other options to consider.

Those options included an intraoral appliance to help reshape her jaw, along with nose cones that she would insert in her nasal passages at night. The soft, flexible cones were designed to help her breathe through her nose, rather than through her mouth. Her mother was concerned that the nose cones might somehow damage her daughter's pretty little nose. But I assured her that the cones were designed only to be worn during sleep to help Elena breathe, and they were to be removed in the morning, at which point Elena's nose would regain its shape.

Ultimately, Elena's mother was convinced to let Elena try the cones for a couple of nights. "Just see how they feel," I told her.

Two days later, her mother reported that Elena's dark circles were gone and that her daughter felt great.

I also gave Elena a series of Myobrace appliances. Myobrace pre-orthodontic treatment addresses issues relating to breathing and swallow dysfunction, allowing patients to reach their genetic potential.

They decided to delay Elena's orthodontic treatment and, before long, Elena's jaw had moved forward, and her tongue thrust, which was threatening to alter the shape of her teeth, was gone.

She was already a pretty girl before the treatment, but afterward, she was even prettier. Plus, she felt great, and the treatment was easy to do.

A number of structural and functional preventive measures can be taken to help a child's facial structure develop in the early years. That early development is key to a future free of TMJ and sleep-disordered breathing problems. Let me explain how.

IN THE BEGINNING

Babies are born with a sucking reflex, or a natural ability to suckle, which develops when they are still inside their mother's womb. When they use that reflex to breastfeed during the first six months of life, it stimulates proper development of the jaw, the nasal passages, and the swallowing reflex.[23] The upper and lower jaws grow forward to the appropriate length, allowing for the rest of the facial structure to properly develop. Imagine the position of your tongue and teeth when you suck on a straw; your tongue touches the back of your top front teeth as you suck. In that position, with the mouth closed, breathing must be done through the nose. That's how the nasal passages are developed as a result of breastfeeding.

So, breastfeeding for the first six months is important for proper development of the skull and craniocervical mandibular area (the neck and lower jaw),[24] nasal breathing, swallowing, and tongue posture. These areas contain a complex network of tissues, blood vessels, and nerves that are easily affected by compression disorders.

Unlike breastfeeding, bottle feeding does not allow for proper development of these areas of the body. In fact, bottle feeding can sometimes lead to severe malformations, especially when parents enlarge the hole in the nipple of the bottle to allow more liquid to flow through. The child must then push their tongue forward to control the flow of liquid in order to keep from drowning. That leads to the development of bad habits, such as tongue-forward posture and a lower resting tongue, neither of which stimulate the upper jaw to grow.

23   D. C. James and B. Dobson, "Position of the American Dietetic Association: Promoting and Supporting Breastfeeding," *Journal of the American Dietetic Association* 105 (2005): 810–18.

24   S. Takahashi, S. Ono, and T. Kuroda, "Effect of Wearing Cervical Headgear on Tongue Pressure," *Journal of Orthodontics* 27 (June 2000): 163–67; K. M. Westover, M.K. DiLoreto, and T.R. Shearer, "The Relationship of Breastfeeding to Oral Development and Dental Concerns," *Journal of American Society of Dentistry for Children* 56, no. 2, (March-April 1989): 140–43.

ORAL CARE FOR BABIES

- From day one, clean the baby's mouth with wet gauze wrapped around your finger.

- At three to four months, a baby can start to identify different tastes. At this age, in addition to breastfeeding, a natural juice may be given in a bottle once or twice a day. No citrus juices.

- At five to six months of life, a child can eat mashed fruits. Avoid foods with sugar, corn syrup, fat, and added coloring agents and preservatives.

- By age two, a child can chew all kinds of food.

PROBLEMS FROM BOTTLE FEEDING

Poor tongue and facial structure development from bottle feeding can lead to a range of problems, including tongue thrust, which I have discussed previously. Tongue thrust occurs as the result of an incorrect position of the tongue during swallowing. Tongue thrust can create a space or gap between the upper and lower teeth and lead to a malformed bite and mouth breathing. Mouth breathing can cause a range of problems, from cavities (because saliva helps protect the teeth) and crooked teeth, to bad breath and gum decay.

People who breathe through their mouths also have smaller airways, which can cause sleep-disordered breathing. Imagine trying to sleep all night with your mouth open. Chances are you'll wake up repeatedly and wake in the morning with a dry mouth and headache. Poor sleep patterns in children can disrupt the body's ability to make growth hormone, which can lead to developmental problems. Enlarged tonsils and adenoids can lead to mouth breathing, which, as I mentioned, may require surgery—a fairly common procedure in young children for airway obstruction.

Another way to correct mouth breathing caused by a narrow jaw is to use expansion appliances to widen it, which will also help open the nasal passages.

Mouth breathers also have increased muscle activity on the buccinators, or muscles in the cheeks. That can lead to soreness after a night of bruxing or clenching and grinding.[25]

One of the major problems with mouth breathing is that it can affect the positions of the teeth. When a person breathes through their mouth, their tongue positions incorrectly while swallowing—it pushes forward, through the front teeth.[26] That can lead to tongue thrust and an open bite, which I discussed earlier.[27] Increased tongue forces can also change the shape of the lower jaw. A tongue thrust when swallowing brings the upper front teeth forward, while preventing the lower teeth from erupting, or coming into the mouth, completely.[28]

THE ERUPTION OF TEETH

The forces delivered by the muscles of the cheeks, lips, and tongue affect the positions of the teeth and the size and shape of the jaw.[29]

25   U. Thüer, R. Sieber, and B. Ingervall, "Cheek and Tongue Pressures in the Molar Areas and the Atmospheric Pressure in the Palatal Vault in Young Adults," *European Journal of Orthodontics* 21, no. 3 (June 1999): 299–309.

26   S. Takahashi et al., "Effect of Changes in the Breathing Mode and Body Position on Tongue Pressure with Respiratory-Related Oscillations," *American Journal of Orthodontics and Dentofacial Orthopedics* 115 (1999): 239–46.

27   Thüer et al., "Cheek and Tongue Pressures in the Molar Areas."

28   Takahashi et al., "Effect of Wearing Cervical Headgear."

29   Thüer et al., "Cheek and Tongue Pressures in the Molar Areas."

The positions of the posterior (back) teeth are affected by the forces of the tongue in the cheek and the incisors (front teeth) are affected by the forces from the muscles of the lips and the tip of the tongue. Increased forces from the cheek muscles with no counteracting force on the inside surfaces creates a triangular arch, which as I mentioned, was Elena's problem.[30]

The impact on the teeth during the act of chewing causes tension on the alveolar bone, which holds the teeth, helping it to develop.[31] Activities such as chewing, sucking, kissing, and whistling involve the muscles of the head, neck, and lower jaws. During these activities, the forces on the jaws affect the shape and size of the bones of the head.[32]

When the facial structure and tongue do not develop correctly, then the eruption (growing in) of teeth is affected.

Incisors typically erupt in the mouth first, usually in the lower jaw. Incisors are those narrow-edged teeth in front of the mouth responsible for cutting food. These commonly erupt at around six months. When the incisors erupt, then the tongue repositions from the roof of the mouth into the lower jaw as the sucking reflex evolves into the chewing mode. Around age two, the child has a full set of teeth, allowing him or her to chew food.

---

30   J.R.C. Mew, "The Postural Basis of Malocclusion: A Philosophical Overview," *American Journal of Orthodontics & Dentofacial Orthopedics* 126, no. 6 (December 2004): 729–38.

31   A. Bresin, S. Kiliaridis, and K.G. Strid, "Effect of Masticatory Function on the Internal Bone Structure in the Mandible of the Growing Rat," *European Journal of Oral Sciences* 107, no. 1 (February 1999): 35–44.

32   H. M. Frost, "A 2003 Update of Bone Physiology and Wolff's Law for Clinicians," *The Angle Orthodontist* 74, no. 1 (February 2004): 3–15; Thüer et al., "Cheek and Tongue Pressures in the Molar Areas."

Ideally, the developing child chews on both sides of the mouth equally, moving their mouth side to side as they chew.[33] However, sometimes a child chews on one side of the mouth or the other. That can indicate a development issue—the jaw may not be developing on both sides, the teeth may not be coming in correctly on one side, the bottom front teeth may be covering the top teeth (instead of the top covering the bottom). If the child purposely chews on one side more than the other—maybe because of pain in the mouth from a cavity—that can cause one side of the jaw to develop more than the other because the act of chewing actually stimulates bone growth.

A GOOD BITE

By age four, children's chewing and swallowing patterns are set. They can open and close their mouth, and move their jaws side to side, allowing them to eat hard and semi-hard foods. If their bite is developing correctly, then their primary teeth, those incisors that erupted first, are beginning to show wear and there is diastema, or spacing, in between them. Although parents are often concerned by that spacing, it's actually a good thing—it indicates that the child's permanent teeth are more likely to erupt without crowding.

Again, chewing helps stimulate bone growth. It does that by creating forces on the ligaments in the teeth. Those ligaments are attached to the jawbone and stimulating them helps the mandible and maxilla (upper and lower jaws) to form.[34] In addition to being

---

33 P. Planas, *Rehabilitation Neuro-Occlusal (RNO)* (Barcelona: Masson-Salvat Odontalogia, 1994); G. P. Neto, R.M. Puppin-Rontani, and R.C. Garcia, "Changes in the Masticatory Cycle After Treatment of Posterior Crossbite in Children Aged 4 to 5 Years," *American Journal of Orthodontics and Dentofacial Orthopedics* 131 (2007): 464–72.

34 V. Krishnan and Z. Davidovitch, "Cellular, Molecular, and Tissue-Level Reaction to Orthodontic Force," *American Journal of Orthodontics and Dentofacial*

nutritious, eating crunchy foods, such as apples and carrots, can stimulate bone growth.

However, when chewing is uneven, then on the non-chewing side, the mandible condyle (the back side of the jawbone) grows downward and forward. Lack of stimulation also causes the teeth to come in unevenly.

By age seven to eight, any malocclusions, or malformed bites, are fully set. That's why treatment of malocclusions must take place early in a child's development in order to address issues that can occur later.

FUNCTION FIRST, THEN FORM

It is imperative to correct any altered oral functions—chewing, swallowing, speech, and breathing—before straightening teeth with orthodontics. As I mentioned, the tongue is a very strong muscle, able to exert up to 500 grams of pressure on the front teeth to push them out of place. No matter how much those teeth are closed together with braces, the tongue can still push them apart once orthodontic treatment is finished. That can ultimately lead to crooked teeth and other problems.[35] That's why people who don't wear a retainer after orthodontic treatment often relapse. When all the functional components of the facial structure are corrected first, then there is no tongue thrust, no relapse after braces are removed, and no long-term need to wear retainers.

In other words, it's best to find the cause of the malocclusion or misalignment of teeth before initiating orthodontic treatment.

Orthopedics 129, no. 4 (April 2006): 469,e 1–32, https://doi.org/10.1016/j.ajodo.2005.10.007

35   Thüer et al., "Cheek and Tongue Pressures in the Molar Areas."

Sometimes the problems in the mouth may be caused by nutritional deficiencies, as Dr. Weston Price, a dentist from Cleveland, Ohio, discovered. He traveled the world to study humans in isolated settings and what he found with groups such as the Aborigines of Australia is that they had beautiful, straight, decay-free teeth. They also had healthy, nutrient-dense diets. In fact, he found that the parents' diet even affected teeth. In a pair of Samoan boys, he found that one born of parents with a good diet had a mouthful of beautiful teeth, while the other, born of parents who had turned away from their native diet, had crowded teeth and was more apt to have decay.[36] This touches on the subject of the next chapter, which is how the foods people eat and their genetic makeup affect the health of the mouth.

Which of these babies do you think is breathing correctly?

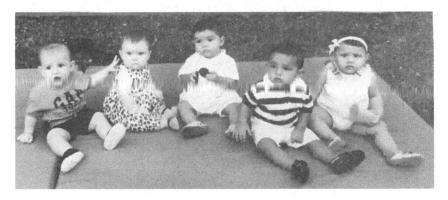

Image care of Dr. German Ramirez.
The baby in the middle is the only one who is breathing through the nose. We can see this as his mouth is closed and his facial muscles are relaxed. Babies number 1, 4, and 5 are breathing through their mouths. Baby number 2 is sucking in her lower lip and has a distressed look on her face.

---

36   "Weston A. Price, DDS," *The Weston A. Price Foundation*, January 1, 2000, accessed April 30, 2018, www.westonaprice.org/health-topics/nutrition-greats/weston-a-price-dds.

CHAPTER 7

NUTRITION AND EPIGENETICS—THE ROLE OF A DEFLAMING DIET IN TMJ AND GOOD SLEEP

"Let food be thy medicine and medicine be thy food."

—HIPPOCRATES

Although patients often understand the role that diet plays in their overall health, many are surprised to find out that factors such as what their mother ate, or what their family traditionally eats, may have also played a role in their issues with breathing-related sleep disorders and TMJ. That happens when outside stimulus detected by the body causes modifications at the cellular level, something known as *epigenetics*.

Epigenetics is defined as functionally relevant changes to the genome (gene) that do not involve the DNA sequence. The genome is the complete set of genetic material in the body's cells—that includes the DNA and all the genes. DNA (or deoxyribonucleic acid) is the "code" within each cell that instructs the body how to grow, develop, function, and reproduce. And genes essentially determine hereditary traits—they transfer physical and functional characteristics from parents to children.

When changes occur in the genome, they may only be temporary and last through division of the cell or only for the duration of the cell's life. Or those changes may be permanent and affect multiple generations. The general consensus definition of *epigenetic trait* is that it is a "stably heritable phenotype resulting from changes in chromosome without alterations in the DNA sequence."[37] In other words, an epigenetic trait is a recognizable and permanent change in the microstructure of the cell that has not affected the underlying DNA sequence. While epigenetics can change the structure of the cell without damaging the DNA, damage to the DNA can cause changes to the epigenome.

HERITABLE TRAITS

When changes to the epigenome are permanent, they can be passed on from generation to generation. Known as *transgenerational epigenetic inheritance*, these changes or markers can be acquired on the DNA of one generation and passed on through genes to the next generation.

In humans, studies have found that identical twins with the same genome vary greatly in their susceptibility to disease because of epigenetic differences occurring over time. While twins may be indistinguishable in their gene expression and profile early in life, older twins have been found to have significant differences in their epigenetic profile.[38]

---

37 S. L. Berger, et al., "An Operational Definition of Epigenetics," *Genes & Development* 23 (2009): 781–83.

38 M. F. Fraga, et al., "Epigenetic Difference Arise During the Lifetime of Monozygolic Twins," *Proceedings of the National Academy of Sciences, USA*, vol. 102, no.

Behaviors, including those that are addictive, can be inherited because of epigenetics. You likely have seen this yourself: Maybe a friend who has an alcohol and gambling problem came from a family in which the parents also had alcohol and gambling problems. Addiction is a disorder of the brain's reward systems. It occurs over time from chronically high levels of exposure to an addictive stimulus, such as morphine, cocaine, alcohol, nicotine, or gambling. When changes to the genome occur as a result, that epigenetic inheritance may become transgenerational.[39]

Emotional experiences can also be passed on. Studies in mice have also shown that conditional fears can be inherited from either parent. For example, mice were conditioned to fear the strong smell of acetophenone when it was accompanied by an electric shock. But even after the shock was no longer given, the mice learned to fear the smell of acetophenone. Remarkably, this display of fear to the scent was passed on to the offspring, even though the offspring had never experienced the electric shock. These epigenetic changes lasted several generations without reintroduction of the shock.[40]

Early childhood experiences can influence a brain for a lifetime. But exposure to detrimental stimuli even earlier, particularly in the womb and shortly after birth, can also increase susceptibility to diseases and other problems by modifying the epigenome. For instance, when a mother has a stressful pregnancy, that stress transfers to the baby. If a mother experiences a reaction to a certain

---

30 (July 26, 2005): 10604–09.

39 R. J. Robison and E. J. Nestler, "Transcriptional and Epigenetic Mechanisms of Addiction," *Nature Reviews Neuroscience* 12, no. 11, (October 12, 2011): 623–37; F. M. Vassoler and G. Sadri-Vakili, "Mechanisms of Transgenerational Inheritance of Addictive-Like Behaviors," *Neuroscience* 264 (April 2014): 198–206.

40 M. Szyf, "Lamarek Revisited. Epigenetic Inheritance of Ancestral Odor Fear Conditioning," *Nature Neuroscience* 17 (2014): 2–4.

substance—a chemical, a scent, a certain food—the child may adopt that same reaction.

Childhood abuse and early trauma also leave epigenetic marks on genes. Maltreatment and extreme stress not only cause immediate harm and potentially impede a child's development, but they can also cause dysfunction to the metabolic and immune systems. That can lead to long-term, chronic, physical and mental health problems ranging from obesity, cardiovascular disease, and cancer to depression and suicide, alcohol abuse, and risky or violent behavior.[41] Researchers have observed striking differences in epigenetic profiles when comparing the brains of people who experienced childhood abuse and committed suicide later in life, with the brains of people who did not experience such childhood trauma and later also committed suicide.[42]

But good behaviors can also be passed on. For instance, the amount of nurturing shown to a baby not only influences the type of nurturer that he or she will become but also affects the way the child handles independence and stress—ultimately determining his or her personality as an adult. Researchers at McGill University found that rat pups that were frequently groomed by their mothers in the first weeks were less fearful and handled stress better than did the ones that were ignored by their parents.[43]

Exercise can also result in changes to the epigenetic marks in muscle and fatty tissue. That can explain why a mother who exercises during pregnancy will bear a child with less fat.

---

41   R. Zhao, "Child Abuse Leaves Epigenetic Marks," *National Human Genome Research Institute*, accessed November 2, 2017, www.genome.gov/27554258.

42   P. McGowan, et al., "Epigenetic Regulation of the Glucocorticoid Receptor in Human Brain Associates with Childhood Abuse," *Nature Neuroscience* 12 (2009): 342–348.

43   "Lick Your Rats," *Learn. Genetics*, accessed November 2, 2017, http://learn. genetics.utah.edu/content/epigenetics/rats.

THE ROLE OF FOOD

Genetic studies today have found evidence that the human race is still evolving and through natural selection, genes continue to impact the changes that occur in the body over time. The food people eat is also impacting human evolution and will determine what humans of the future will be like.[44]

Methionine is an amino acid that enters the body through proteins in the food you eat. Your body uses it to form proteins in the body, and it is the precursor (through the methionine cycle) of the sulfur-containing amino acid homocysteine. Amino acids are the building blocks of proteins. When proteins break down, their building blocks collapse, and elevated levels of amino acids like homocysteine may be found in the bloodstream. Excess homocysteine in the blood increases the risk of heart disease, high cholesterol, depression, and Alzheimer's. Homocysteine must be methylated, or joined with methyl-related nutrients, to convert back to methionine. Exercising at least three times per week can lower your risk of elevated levels of homocysteine, as can eating foods rich in folates.

I've been talking throughout the book about the damaging effects of inflammation. Foods such as sugar, dairy products, and gluten can cause inflammation and weight gain all over the body, even in the fingers. When there is excess fat in the neck, it can put more pressure on the airway. If the airway is already small, then the problem worsens with excess weight.

A deflaming diet reduces inflammation all over the body and helps with weight loss, as well.

---

44   B. Handwerk, "How Cheese, Wheat and Alcohol Shaped Human Evolution," *Smithsonian.com*, March 13, 2018, www.smithsonianmag.com/science-nature/how-cheese-wheat-and-alcohol-shaped-human-evolution-180968455.

Children, especially, consume a lot of sugar, milk, and other foods that they may actually be allergic to. Sugar is the worst—it causes inflammation everywhere, including in the nasal passages. When the nasal airway is inflamed, it becomes much easier to breathe through the nose. That can cause a person to develop a bad habit of breathing through the mouth. When that happens, the lower jaw is set back and downward, which can lead to poor tongue position and poor swallowing habits. All of these contribute to sleep issues, a narrowing of the arch, and crowding of teeth.

Sugar, milk, and wheat are also soft foods, so the jaws muscles don't get a workout to develop forward properly. As I mentioned in the previous chapter, crunchy foods like apples can stimulate bone growth. In children, apples are cut up to make the pieces smaller for the child to eat. But a better way to help the child is to give them larger pieces or whole apples that they can bite into. That act of biting into a full apple forces the lower jaw forward, which helps with development and also opens the airway to pull in more air. But with mushier food such as applesauce, the chewing motion is up and down; the lower jaw is not brought forward, so the airway stays small.

I often tell patients to chew on foods such as beef jerky; chew on both sides of the mouth can help the jaws to develop properly. A jaw that develops too narrowly or with a bad bite can potentially help avoid TMJ and sleep problems.

THE ROLE OF ENVIRONMENT AND DIET

Exposure to environmental contamination by endocrine-disrupting chemicals can leave an imprint that is passed down to generations.[45] One such chemical is bisphenol A (BPA)—an additive in some plastics that has been linked to cancer and other diseases—which can make epigenetic modifications. Studies in rats have also demonstrated that exposure during adolescence to THC, the addictive compound in cannabis, can predispose future offspring to heroin addiction. Here again, it changes the epigene, not the actual gene.

Diet can also have a significant impact on changes to the epigenome. Several studies also show that a poor or high-fat diet is detrimental to health across several generations.[46] So what the mother eats when she is pregnant can affect the cells of the fetus.

Studies of humans whose ancestors survived through periods of starvation in Sweden and the Netherlands suggest that the effects of famine on epigenetics and health can pass through at least three generations. One study of Swedish historical records showed that men who had experienced famine before puberty were less likely to have grandsons with heart disease or diabetes than were men who had plenty to eat.[47]

Conversely, a study in 2008 showed that exposing mice brains to just six hours of high blood sugar led to epigenetic changes that increased the risk of vascular damage. These changes lasted for six days, indicating long-term damage after just a short blast of sugar.

---

45 I. Weaver et al., "Epigenetic Programming by Maternal Behavior," *Nature Neuroscience* 7, (2004): 847–88.

46 J. A. McKay and J. C. Mathers, "Diet-Induced Epigenetic Changes and Their Implications for Health," *Acta Physiologica* (Oxford) 202, no. 2 (June 2011): 103–118.

47 G. Kaati, L. R. Bygren, and S. Edvinsson, "Cardiovascular and Diabetes Mortality Determined by Nutrition During Parents' and Grandparents' Slow-Growth Period," *European Journal of Human Genetics* 10, no. 11 (2002): 682–88.

One study found that a low-carbohydrate diet had neuroprotective benefits, providing epigenetic suppression of toxic oxidative stress.[48] Oxidative stress is essentially an imbalance in the body's ability to prevent cell damage. Calorie-restrictive diets also seem to offer this benefit. Therefore, choosing meals lower in carbohydrates and calories improves brain cells' ability to fight off damage, leading to healthier brains.

Surprisingly, US dietary guidelines recommend getting 65 percent of daily calories from carbohydrate sources. But since carbs are converted into sugar as soon as they are digested, that is a dietary plan destined to harm DNA.

A study of the effects of diet on rats found epigenetic changes passed down from both the father and the mother may have negative consequences for offspring. Male rats fed a high-fat diet generated female offspring with a diabetes-like condition, although these offspring were given a normal diet.

The good news is that, unlike genes, which only can be altered through complex gene therapies, epigenetic marks are reversible and can respond to environmental changes or drug treatment.

Reversing the Damage

Most patients' health issues are directly related to their diets. The typical Western diet is filled with refined carbohydrates and animal proteins and does not include many inflammation-reducing Omega 3s. Omega 3s are fatty acids, which are good for the body. A study published in 1995 found that people who ate two meals of fatty fish per month, such as anchovy, mackerel, and salmon, experienced a 30 percent reduction in cardiac arrest. Four fatty fish meals a month

---

48   P. Sassone-Corsi, "Physiology. When metabolism and epigenetics converge," *Science* 339, no. 6116 (January 2013): 148–50.

were associated with a 50 percent reduction in cardiac arrest. Omega 6s, on the other hand, which come from vegetable oil and other foods, should be avoided.

OMEGA 3 FOODS

- Fish: anchovy, mackerel, salmon, sardines

- Nuts and seeds: walnuts, flax seeds, chia seeds

- Navy beans and soybeans

- Vegetables: spinach and brussels sprouts

Fortunately, there are substances capable of undoing DNA damage. An epigenetic diet, for instance, can maximize the health of DNA. Foods such as broccoli, turmeric, green tea, and resveratrol (found in red wine), have demonstrated the ability to slow or reverse damage to the DNA. The chemicals in these foods may prevent cancer formation, decrease fat cells, and lower inflammation.[49]

Foods that improve epigenetics are rich in folate (vitamin B9). These include citrus fruits, strawberries, and leafy green vegetables, and those foods rich in vitamin B12, such as fish, meat, milk, and eggs. Certain nutrients produce methylation, the process I mentioned earlier. Methyl-related nutrients include folates, vitamin B12, and vitamin B6—these change the body chemistry and help rid the body of chemicals, lowering the risk of breast, colon, and pancreatic cancer, according to the National Cancer Institute.

---

49 T. Maeda et al., "The Correlation Between the Telomeric Parameters and the Clinic Laboratory Data in Patients with Brain Infarction and Metabolic Disorders," *The Journal of Nutrition, Health & Aging* 14, no. 9 (November 2010): 793–97; X. Cui et al., "Resveratrol Suppresses Colitis and Colon Cancer Associated with Colitis," *Cancer Prevention Research* 3, no. 4 (April 2010): 549–59.

Foods rich in folates: garbanzo (chickpeas) and pinto beans, lentils, spinach, avocado, asparagus, beets

Foods rich in vitamin B12: fish, poultry, meat, eggs, dairy

Foods rich in vitamin B6: poultry, fish, fortified cereals, beans, dark leafy greens, oranges, cantaloupe, and papayas

Dr. Stephen Sinatra recommends the Pan-Asian Modified Mediterranean diet. The key to this diet is the consumption of essential fatty acids (EFAs), which cannot be manufactured by the body. EFAs penetrate layers of cholesterol plaque, soothing inflammation in blood vessels and preventing blood-clotting deposits from lining coronary arteries. EFAs can also prevent spasms of the coronary blood vessels and the rupture of the plaque.

The Pan-Asian Modified Mediterranean diet, or PAMM diet, recommended by Sinatra includes:

- vegetables such as asparagus, broccoli and kale, brussels sprouts, and spinach

- onions and garlic

- proteins rich in EFAs, such as eggs and wild cold-water fish (salmon and anchovies)

- fruits such as strawberries, blueberries, raspberries, cherries, pears, apples, plums, and peaches

- nuts such as seed nuts, walnuts, almonds, and flax seed

- as many fresh herbs as possible

Foods to be avoided include:

- any food cooked in a factory

- refined flour or sugar contained in breads, bagels, and biscuits, crackers, cookies, and chips

- fruit juices (high in sugar)

- starchy vegetables, such as potatoes, carrots, peas, and corn

- cooking oils such as corn, safflower, soy, and canola

The PAMM diet can also reduce inflammation, which causes irritation leading to swelling in the body's tissues and joints. When it comes to problems of the jaw and mouth and nasal breathing, inflammation is the primary culprit. By controlling harmful inflammation, you can reduce or eliminate illness.

One of the causes of chronic inflammation is a syndrome known as "leaky gut."

What Is Leaky Gut?

More than two thousand years ago, Hippocrates, the father of modern medicine, said, "All disease begins in the gut." Today, that statement still rings true.

In his book *Heal Your Leaky Gut: The Hidden Cause of Many Chronic Diseases*, Dr. David Brownstein explains how environmental toxins, bacteria, processed foods, stress, or medications (prescribed and over-the-counter) can irritate your gut. These irritants can cause tiny pinpricks in the lining of the small intestine, and as a result, undigested food, bacteria, and toxins can leak through the intestinal wall and enter the bloodstream. This leakage compromises absorption of nutrients that nourish the body and give it energy.

Besides poor nutrition absorption, when bacteria and toxins escape the intestines and enter the bloodstream, they cause widespread inflammation. That inflammation can lead to the immune system attacking the body itself, which can be the root cause of chronic illnesses.

When normal digestion is affected, gas, bloating, acid reflux, and heartburn may occur. According to Dr. Leo Galland, director of the Foundation for Integrated Medicine, the following symptoms are signs that may indicate leaky gut:

- chronic diarrhea, constipation, gas, or bloating

- nutritional deficiencies

- poor immune system

- headaches, brain fog, memory loss

- excessive fatigue

In my practice, we go over a deflaming diet with patients at each visit as part of the nutrition piece of treatment. We base our recommendations off of *The DeFlame Diet: DeFlame Your Diet, Body, and Mind* by Dr. David Seaman. The goal is to help patients to better understand how to reduce a chronic inflammatory state with diet and nutritional supplements, such as cutting out sugars, trans fats, and flour, and adding anti-inflammatory vegetables.

Here are some of the items we discuss:

- **Wheat**. Research has shown that consumption of modern wheat can trigger autoimmune diseases, such as diabetes, multiple sclerosis, and arthritis.[50] Modern-day wheat grows on plants that are 18 to 24 inches tall versus the 4.5-foot-tall plants in the past, which reduces the quality of the grain.

- **Sugar**. Added sugar is the worst ingredient in diets. Sugar can increase insulin resistance in the body and may be linked to fatty liver as well as diabetes type 2. Perhaps

---

50   Dr. William Davis, cardiologist and author, talks extensively about the problems with wheat in the diet in his *Wheat Belly* books.

the worst culprits are sugary drinks, which do not satiate because the brain doesn't register them as food. Since the calories in these drinks are not compensated for by eating less food, they add empty calories to the diet. Fruit juices contain antioxidants as well as vitamins, but they're basically full of sugar, so drink juices sparingly.

- **Agave** is also often considered to be a healthy alternative to sugar. However, it is high in fructose, which is not good for you.

  □ **Special note:** Alternatives to sugar may include stevia, a sweetener without calories that has been used for medicinal purposes in South America, or Xylitol, a non-inflammatory sweetener that is as sweet as sugar with two-third of sugar's calories. It reduces the risk of dental cavities.

- **Refined vegetable oils** are high in omega-6 fatty acid. These are sensitive to oxidation and cause increased oxidative stress in the body. They have been linked to an increased risk in cancer. Alternatives may be coconut oil, ghee butter, or extra virgin olive oil.

- **Cakes and cookies**. These are typically made with refined flour, fats, and sugar, which are extra calories the body doesn't need and unhealthy ingredients that can cause inflammation.

- **Junk foods**. These foods are often high in sugar and cornstarch, and low in healthy nutrients.

Nutritional support can also include a range of supplements to help with healing. These include:

- An iron-free multivitamin

- Magnesium (to calm)

- Omega-3 (for heart health)

- Vitamin K (for stronger bones)

- Probiotic (healthy gut bacteria)

- Coenzyme Q10 (for joint health)

- Turmeric (to reduce inflammation)

It's important to understand the roles that epigenetics and nutrition play in reducing inflammation and healing patients. Focusing on the nutritional component, combined with appliance therapy and other treatments used by the TMJ & Sleep Therapy Centre of North Texas and referral partners, can help make you feel whole again.

CHAPTER 8

IT'S NOT ALL IN
YOUR HEAD

"The first step in solving a problem is to recognize that it does exist."

—ZIG ZIGLAR

If you've been to doctor after doctor and still are not getting answers to the problems that are plaguing you, maybe it's time to visit the TMJ & Sleep Therapy Centre of North Texas. Too often, patients are told a problem is "all in their head," but as a patient myself, I know that the problems are very, very real.

TMJ and sleep disorders are often connected, and they can result in a wide range of symptoms that seem disconnected. Headaches, snoring, body aches and pains, and malformed teeth are just some of the symptoms that may ultimately stem from TMJ and sleep-disordered breathing and sleep apnea.

Unfortunately, many people seek help but don't get answers. Or, they get answers for part of the problem, but then that treatment causes other problems.

Today, there are oral appliance treatments that can resolve TMJ and sleep issues, but these are just some of the treatment options that we offer at the TMJ & Sleep Therapy Centre of Texas.

Again, treatments options include:

- **Appliances** that decompress to address either TMJ only, or both TMJ and sleep-disordered breathing or sleep apnea. Depending on the appliance and the patient's need, these are either worn only during the day or are part of a three-appliance therapy to reduce inflammation while helping to prevent grinding at night.

- **Exercises** to help train and build the facial structures, and to help better pace breathing.

- **Anti-inflammatories** such as nasal sprays, NSAIDs, and natural muscle relaxants such as spices, supplements, and teas.

- **Phase II orthodontics** for patients who need additional help correcting malformations.

- **Cold laser** to reduce inflammation, relieve pain, and for some patients, loosen the jaw.

- **CPAP** for sleep apnea. Although not prescribed in our offices, CPAP helps sufferers of sleep apnea and can be used in conjunction with an appliance as part of hybrid treatment for OSA.

At the TMJ & Sleep Therapy Centre of Texas, we look at everything in order to properly diagnose the issue. Every patient undergoes a comprehensive exam that starts with a deep dive into their medical history to help us better understand lifestyle, pains they've been experiencing, and diagnosis and treatment from other providers.

The medical history is followed by a comprehensive exam that includes palpating or pressing on the muscles of the head, neck, and cheeks to check for tenderness. When there is TMJ pain, the muscles involved in clenching and grinding can be very tender. If we palpate the muscle or the joint in front of the ear and the patient expresses that there is pain, then we know they may have TMJ.

We also look at the position of the head compared to the shoulders. When there is a breathing issue, then often a person will position their head forward without realizing it, because that opens the airway. Every inch the head is forward of the shoulders adds ten pounds of pressure on the neck. When that happens, it can cause pain in the neck and shoulders. That's how breathing issues can lead to neck pain.

After the visual and physical exams, we run a number of other tests to help arrive at the right diagnosis. Some of those include:

- Photos to assess a patient's face, head, and neck symmetry.

- Palpation of head and neck.

- X-rays, scans, and 3-D imaging to look at anatomic changes inside the mouth and in the jaw, head, and neck.

- Motor nerve reflex testing, an orthopedic neurological test to look specifically for TMJ. Motor nerve reflex testing includes the light/dark scratch, and posture tests to look for injury or dystrophy in the body's nervous system.

Once testing is complete and a diagnosis is made, patients undergo comprehensive and customized treatment based on their individual needs. That treatment may include orthodontics, chiropractic, sleep therapy, or other solutions first, depending on the patient's needs.

Remember: If you're plagued with problems that don't seem to have a solution, don't let anyone tell you, "It's all in your head." If you or someone you know is experiencing the symptoms of TMJ or sleep-disordered breathing, reach out to us at the TMJ & Sleep Therapy Centre of North Texas.

TMJ SYMPTOMS

- Pain in lower jawbone

- Inability to open the mouth widely

- Fatigue of jaw muscles

- Problems with chewing

- Swelling at the jaw joints

ADULT SLEEP APNEA SIGNS AND SYMPTOMS:

- Loud Snoring

- Excessive daytime sleepiness

- Morning headaches

- Teeth grinding

- Dental changes

- Depression

- Diabetes

- Obesity

- Heartburn and GERD

CHILDREN SLEEP APNEA SIGNS AND SYMPTOMS:

- Snoring, mouth-breathing

- Restlessness, odd sleep positions

- Bedwetting

- Night terrors

- Headaches

- Teeth grinding

Don't wait, take action now, because the issues you are having today can turn into lifelong problems.

GETTING TO THE SOURCE OF THE PROBLEM

My struggles with TMJ began in my teenage years and persisted well into adulthood. In 2014, I was referred to Dr. Krish by my dentist after having clenched my jaw so hard on a business trip that I broke a crown. It was on that same trip that I bought a clunky rolling backpack to replace my shoulder bag because of neck, shoulder and lower back pain that I'd been experiencing for some time. At that point, my quality of life was really suffering.

When Dr. Krish suggested that she could correct my TMJ dysfunction (which it turns out was also the source of my neck, shoulder, and back pain) with an oral appliance, I was skeptical. How could this work when jaw surgery had not provided lasting relief? As a last effort, I decided to give it a try. Much to my surprise, Dr. Krish's protocol (which also included cold laser therapy) worked to stop the bruxism and heal the pain that was diminishing my quality of life.

Once my TMJ issues were resolved, Dr. Krish gave me a take-home test for sleep apnea. It turned out that I had severe obstructive sleep apnea, which explained why I awakened at night gasping and never felt rested. Dr. Krish addressed this by making a modification to my oral appliance. Soon, not only was I pain free, but I was also sleeping through the night.

My teenage daughter is now undergoing Myobrace treatment with Dr. Krish to correct her bite and I am pleased to say that she is also experiencing very positive results. Singing is her passion. This treatment is not only helping her teeth to come in straight, it is also improving her breathing, which has had a significant impact on her singing.

The treatment that my family has received from Dr. Krish and her staff has been life changing. I will forever be grateful to her. What I appreciate most about Dr. Krish is that she doesn't just treat symptoms, she uncovers and addresses the root cause. I wish more doctors would take this approach.

—Donna Bailey

RELIEF THE FIRST NIGHT

For at least a decade I was a heavy snorer who would momentarily stop breathing during the night. I never recognized the impact this had on my sleep quality, but it significantly impacted my wife's sleep quality. Amazingly, it wasn't the snoring that interrupted her sleep, it was the silence because that meant I had stopped breathing. Four to six times a night I would go silent and she would wake up, shake me to get me breathing, then rest fairly easy while I snored away.

It took the negative impact on my wife's sleep, and not the negative impact on my own health, to spur me into fixing my problem. For a variety of reasons, CPAP was a solution of last resort for me, and I always want to avoid surgical options. I decided an oral appliance would be the first potential solution I would try, it turned out to be the ideal solution for me.

The snoring and breathing interruption stopped the very first night. Within a week I recognized I no longer felt tired toward the end of the work day. In a year of wearing the device there have been zero stopped breathing occurrences. My predominate sleeping position is on my side and my wife cannot recall any snoring when on my side; there is occa-

sional snoring when I am sleeping on my back. I had a sleep apnea test with the device a couple of months after first use; I passed the test with flying colors!

—James O'Donnell

I WISH I HAD KNOWN SOONER!

My treatment with Dr. Krish began in late September but my suffering with the symptoms of TMJ (popping, locking, and clicking of the jaw, soreness and pain, malalignment of teeth/bite) has been ongoing since the early 1990s. I finished my treatment in December and my only regret is that I didn't know of Dr. Krish sooner. The specialist that I consulted in my early twenties described the course of "treatment" to me, which consisted of essentially filing down my natural tooth structure and rebuilding the teeth in alignment with where the jaw naturally wants to close. I was a college student at the time and didn't have the money needed for treatment. But, even then, I questioned the logic of filing and rebuilding my teeth, as I felt that such extensive dental work would certainly require a fair amount of maintenance through the years. Dr. Krish's treatment restored my jaw to its natural position without doing any work on my teeth or performing any surgical procedures. After one week of treatment, not only had my symptoms improved drastically but my jaw placement was already corrected. I never tried to force it, but that's what it would have taken to get it in the position it was before. I was amazed. One of the best parts of Dr. Krish's treatment is that she explains and visually demonstrates how the problem is multifaceted. It's not just the teeth, the nasal passages, the tongue, the joint, etc., but how they all work together and how it causes problems when they don't work together properly. Her treatment actually made sense to me! The end results were worth the money spent because it's a permanent solution, which is a great alternative to just living with pain and discomfort. I am so thankful that she has chosen to help people who suffer needlessly. I am also thankful that my dentist, Dr. Morris, referred me to her. Last, but definitely not least, I have to mention what a wonderful, caring, friendly, and professional staff she has. I was a little sad when my treatment had concluded because I had gotten to know them so well. What a difference a well-informed, well-trained team of professionals makes!

—Rhonda Powell

CONTACT US

At TMJ & Sleep Therapy Centre of North Texas, we know that the complexity and severity of pain, sleep disorders, and breathing disorders can vary for each patient, and that finding relief for these issues can be frustrating and confusing. But with proper evaluation and diagnosis, the conditions of craniofacial pain, TMJ, sleep apnea, and snoring can be successfully treated.

Our highly trained staff is exclusively dedicated to the comprehensive evaluation for proper diagnosis and implementation of non-invasive treatment therapies. Using state-of-the-art technology and research-based treatment in a caring and friendly environment, we recognize and treat each patient as a unique individual.

Reach out to us at:

TMJ & Sleep Therapy Centre of North Texas
1005 Long Prairie Road, Suite 300
Flower Mound, Texas 75022
972-538-3777
www.krish.com

Printed in the USA
CPSIA information can be obtained
at www.ICGtesting.com
JSHW012041140824
68134JS00033B/3192

9 781599 328836